Yoga Challenge® I

Practice Manual

Hatha Yoga in the Bishnu Ghosh tradition.

Yoga Challenge® I

Practice Manual

Hatha Yoga in the Bishnu Ghosh tradition.

Tony Sanchez

Tony Sanchez Academia de Yoga
Baja California Sur, Mexico
www.tonysanchezyoga.com

Yoga Challenge® I
Practice Manual

Copyright© 2007, Tony Sanchez
Second Edition

All rights reserved.
Printed in the United States of America.
No part of this book may be reproduced,
stored in a retrieval system, or transmitted by any means,
electronic, mechanical, photocopying, recording,
or otherwise, without written permission from the author.

ISBN: 1-4196-2909-3

Editing & Photographs: Sandy Sanchez
Special thanks to Alex Wheeler

To order additional copies, visit
Tony Sanchez Academia de Yoga
www.tonysanchezyoga.com.
or
www.booksurge.com

CONTENTS

PREFACE   !

I. ORIGINS   0
    Myth
    Sages
    Yoga Challenge® I

II. SCIENCE   29
    Science of Yoga
    Science of Practice
    Science of the Body

III. PRACTICE   45
Mind/Body Practice
Yoga Challenge Practice

IV. YOGA CHALLENGE® I   63

Standing Asanas

Breathing Series (part I)   69
1. Standing Deep Breathing

Half Moon Series   72
2. Lateral Half Moon
3. Back Stretch
4. Forward Stretch, Hands-to-Feet
5. Triangle
6. Standing Separate Leg Head-to-Knee

Awkward Series   84
7. Awkward
8. Eagle
9. Standing Head-to-Knee
10. Standing Bow
11. Balancing Stick
12. Splits-in-the-Air
13. Separate-Leg-Stretching
14. Tree

Transition Series   106
14. Finger Stand
15. Lotus Warm-up
16. Shoulder Roll
17. Pelvic Lift
18. Corpse
19. Wind Removing Sit-up

Floor Asanas

Cobra Series — 122
    20. Cobra
    21. Locust
    22. Bow

Half Tortoise Series — 132
    23. Half Tortoise
    24. Camel
    25. Rabbit

Stretching Series — 140
    26. Head-to-Knee
    27. Stretching
    28. Separate-Leg-Stretching
    29. Upward Gas-Removing
    30. Upward Stretching

Abdominal Series — 150
    31. Extended Arms
    32. Interlaced Fingers
    33. Leg Crunch
    34. Crossed Arms
    35. Arms on Floor

Double Sided Series — 156
    36. Cow Face
    37. Spinal Twist
    38. Lateral Spine Twist
    39. Abdominal Twist

Breathing Series (part II) — 166
    40. Blowing Pose (*Kapalabati*)

BIBLIOGRAPHY

*". . . it is never too late to begin
the practice of this yoga system,
for it helps to rebuild the body,
reenergize the mind,
revive lost youth, beauty and strength,
make youth last longer and
repair the damage silently done by
wrong methods of living, and by
disobedience of nature's simple laws;
body and mind are so closely related that
if one is healthy,
the other must also be so."*
                                        Buddha Bose

PREFACE

The second edition of *The Yoga Challenge® I* was written with the student and the teacher in mind. This manual provides enough information to take on the practice of yoga in a safe but challenging way. Emphasis is on utilizing the basic principles of alignment and movement established by physical therapist. These principles include the anatomical or *central* position, the starting point for all poses in the system. They are the basis and foundation of alignment, proper weight distribution and good posture. Use them to measure your progress in flexibility, strength and balance as a result of regular practice.

This manual is a reference for instructors-in-training, practitioners and instructors. Home-practitioners can use it as a step-by-step manual or companion to the Yoga Challenge® I DVD. For practitioners and instructors from other schools of yoga, the asanas are classic Hatha Yoga with technical information that applies to all.

This manual outlines a simple but effective way to practice and teach the *Yoga Challenge® I* for therapeutic and physical wellness. The first step is to take control and responsibility for your own practice and, as an instructor, encourage your students to do the same.

The science of the *Yoga Challenge® I* is in applying the principles and focusing inward to observe and, eventually, understand how the poses work on your body. Each has a unique way in which it stimulates joints, muscles, tendons, ligaments, systems and organs of the body.

Mastery of the poses evolves gradually over time with disciplined practice. Standards of excellence are reached and maintained by following the basic principles that require precision when practicing.

The poses in the *Yoga Challenge® I* are cultural and therapeutic. The sequence is designed to restore and maintain range-of-motion, alignment and proper stimulation to all vital organs and systems which is of utmost importance for a long and healthy life. Regular practice can play a significant role in the prevention of many physical, emotional and mental maladies often generated by unhealthy lifestyle and habits, muscle imbalances, faulty alignment and improper, or lack of exercise.

Although the *Yoga Challenge® I* training program is the ideal way to become an instructor, we realize not everyone is able or inclined to do so. In that case, please do read this manual carefully in order to teach with utmost integrity and in the spirit of the teacher.

Yogis believed that good health and regulated breath developed the clarity of mind to know and fulfill one's purpose in life. Having the clarity of mind to teach yoga for nearly 30 years, I hope that sharing some of what I have learned through my practice, teachings and business in yoga will be helpful to those who have chosen or may choose the same path.

To begin, you must make the commitment to regular, consistent practice. Sometimes it is difficult and frustrating, sometimes it is lonely, but the benefits are all yours.

> *"Faith in the practice of Yoga and in one's own powers to accomplish what others have done before, is of great importance to insure speedy success."*
> Pancham Sinh

"Live each present moment completely and the future will take care of itself."
Yogananda

ORIGINS

*"Quite apart from the charm of the new and
fascination of the half-understood,
there is good cause for yoga to have many adherents.
It offers the possibility of controllable experience and, thus,
satisfies the scientific need for 'facts'; and, besides this,
by reason of its breadth and depth,
its' venerable age, its doctrine and method,
which include every phase of life,
it promises undreamed-of possibilities."*
　　　　　　　　　　　　　　　　Carl G. Jung

Myth

The origin and evolution of the universe, and Vishnu's dream according to the Rudrasamhita and the Matsyamahapurana.

The Beginning

The cosmos and the great dissolution began simultaneously; matter, the elements, the planets, the sun, the moon and the stars were all particles in one big, dark void.

Sat-Brahman (The Absolute)

According to the Vedas, the void was Sat-Brahman, impossible to understand or describe with words. The universe exists because of it, it has no beginning or end.

Origins

Ishvara (Universal-Self, Shiva)

Out of the formless Sat-Brahman a second presence eventually evolved. Ishvara, the Universal-Self, Shiva, the supreme Brahman, pervades everything with its essence.

Shakti (Universal Energy)

Shakti, the universal energy, evolved from Ishvara's essence. She has several manifestations that include Pradhana, Prakrti, Maya, Kalika, Durga and Gunavati. She is the mother of the Buddhi Tattva (cosmic intelligence) and the generating force behind everything in creation. More importantly, Shakti is the mother of the three deities; Rudra, Vishnu and Brahma. Shakti as Maya (the power of creation), together with Kala (time) created Sivaloka, a holy center of bliss that Shiva called the blissful forest.

Vishnu (The Savior)

Shiva and Shakti enjoyed dueling in the blissful forest for an eternity before creating Vishnu from a fragrant nectar secreted from Siva's left side. Vishnu had the power to create everything in the universe, protect it, then let it dissolve and begin a new cycle. Pleased with his creation, Shiva gave Vishnu the Vedas through his nostrils before vanishing with Shakti.

After more than 12,000 years of meditation, Vishnu reached enlightenment. He was delighted but wanted to know more so he continued, forcing himself to exhaustion. He perspired profusely, immersing himself in a pool of the Sat-Brahman in watery form before creating Sesa, the thousand-headed serpent, symbol of infinity, coiled and floating on the divine waters of the cosmos.

Brahma (The Creator)

Vishnu, as Narayana (one residing in water), sleeping in the coils of Sesa, dreamt of a gigantic lotus stalk flowing from his naval that grew to infinity. Within the brilliant colored blossom he saw Shiva and Shakti create Brahma from Siva's right side. Known as the lotus-born god, Brahma is creator of the universe. The lotus is a symbol of re-birth or re-manifestation. Together, Brahma, Vishnu and Shiva represent the three states of consciousness.

Twenty-five Elements of Creation (Tattvas)

Brahma had a vision one day where he saw the five forms of Shiva, containing the 25 elements of creation (tattvas), manifest life. The symbolic forms are associated with gross and subtle elements: organs of action, organs of knowledge, the mind, ego, intellect, nature and the soul.

Name	Form	Organ of Knowledge	Organ of Action	Subtle/Gross Element
Isana	Soul	Ears	Speech	Sound/Ether
Aghora	Intellect	Eye	Feet	Form/Fire
Tatpurusa	Nature	Skin	Hand	Touch/Wind
Vamadeva	Ego	Tongue	Anus	Taste/Water
Sadyojata	Mind	Nose	Regeneration	Smell/Earth

Day of Brahma

Each of Siva's five forms presides over a specific *kalpa*, or day of Brahma, equal to 432,000,000 human years. Vishnu's dream lasts about 100 Brahma years. One year of Brahma has 360 Brahma days, each consisting of 12 million divine years. Vishnu's dream is synonymous with the life of Brahma and consistent with the mythological concept of harmony between the cycles of the human body and the universe.

In the *Shiva Purana,* one kalpa is divided into 14 world cycles called Manvataras, defined by the different ages of the Manu. They are: 1. Svayambhuva, 2. Svarocisa, 3.Uttaa, 4.Tamasa, 5. Raivata, 6. Caksusa, 7. Vaivasvata, 8. Savarni, 9. Raucya, 10. Brahma-Savarni, 11. Dharma-Savarni, 12. Rudra-Sarvani, 13. Deva- Sarvani and 14. Indra-Sarvani.

We currently live in cycle number seven, Vaivasvata Manu.

Dissolution

Minor dissolutions take place at the end of each cycle, concluding with a great dissolution at the end of the fourteenth, and final one. Everything Brahma created will dissolve and merge into his body before he dissolves into the essence of Vishnu to lie dormant for a period of time before beginning the process again.

At the end of Vishnu's 100 Brahma-year dream the greatest of all dissolutions will take place. Everything will be absorbed back into the Sat-Brahman, the infinite black void, before the cycle begins again

Five days of Brahma

It took 18 Brahma days from the first year of his 100-year life to manifest the five forms of Shiva that constitute creation.

1. On the 19th Kalpa known as Svetalohita, Brahma meditated on the Sat-Brahman and saw Shiva incarnate as Sadyojata and manifest sons in the form of the Sat-Brahman. They bestowed on Brahma great wisdom and the power of creation. Sadyojata then manifested the earth.

2. On the 20th Kalpa known as Rakta, Brahma assumed an intense red essence while he meditated on the lotus of his heart and saw Vamadeva dressed in red. Knowing he was an incarnation of Shiva, Brahma bowed with hands joined in reverence and received perfect wisdom and the power to create. Vamadeva manifested water.

3. On the 21st Kalpa, known as the Pitavasas, Brahma assumed a yellow essence and meditated on his heart to see the incarnation of Shiva as the Tat-Purusa, dressed in yellow garments, engrossed in meditation. Before bowing to him Brahma performed the Japa of Siva-Gayatri, the great goddess and Tat-Purusa manifested sons, dressed in yellow, from his sides. They were the instigators of the Yogic path. In the form of nature Tat-Purusa manifested wind.

4. On the 22nd Kalpa, known as Shiva, Brahma was in a state of sorrow. A thousand divine years had passed, the entire universe had become one vast ocean and creation was in a dormant state. In his sorrow he saw Aghora, in the form of a Brahman. His garments, turban and skin were black. and, the four sons that sprang from his sides, all in the form of Shiva, were also black. To assist Brahma with creation, they manifested fire and initiated the great Yoga Ghora.

5. On the 23rd Kalpa, known as Visvarpa (universe formed), Brahma meditated on the Sat-Brahman in his heart and saw Sarasvati, goddess of sound and speech, manifesting herself as the energy of the universe. He then focused his meditation on Shiva and saw before him the form of Isana, who manifested the soul and ether, or space. Realizing he was the last incarnation of Shiva in the scheme of creation, he bowed to him with great reverence. Isana instructed Brahma on the path of good then created four sons with Sarasvati's energy. By means of Yoga his sons imparted virtue and attained the goal of Yoga.

Brahma's children

After manifesting the five forms of Shiva, Brahma practiced austerities and the Vedas were revealed to him. From various parts of his body Brahma then created 10 sons and one daughter known as the Manasas. From his right thumb came Prajapati Daksa, from his breast, Dharma, from his heart, Cupid, from his brows, Anger, from his lips, Greed, from his intellect, Delusion, from his ego, Arrogance, from his throat, Glee, from his eyes, Death, from his hands, Bharata, the sage, and, finally, a daughter, Angaja.

After creating the Manasas, Brahma resumed severe penance by lifting his arms over his head like a Sadhu. Eventually, he saw Vishnu in the form of a Yogi along with Kapila, teacher of Sankya, singing praises to him. Feeling encouraged by what he heard Brahma used his yogic powers to create the three realms (heaven, earth and the underworld), along with three more sons. The first was created to meditate on truth, eternity and emancipation, the second was dedicated to the study of the *Vedas*, and the third studied the philosophy of Sankhya and became known as Bhurbhuvah, knower of Sankhya.

After creating the 25 elements (bhutas) of creation, the Manasas, the three realms and more sons, Brahma was tired but still not satisfied. He confided in the goddess Gayatri who manifested a young girl, Satarupa, from half of his body to help him carry on with creation. Enchanted by her beauty, Brahma fell madly in love with his daughter, unable to keep his eyes off of her.

Five heads of Brahma

Satarupa, however, was very shy and tried to evade Brahma's gaze. In an effort to follow her every move without disturbing her, Brahma created three heads around his existing one, each facing a different direction. When she ascended to heaven with the Manasas to escape him, he grew a fifth head on top of the other four to look up. Having surrendered to Cupid's spell of love and lust, Brahma lost his great powers acquired through penance and meditation. He directed his sons to carry on with the work of creating while he pursued Satarupa.

Daksa Prajapati: father of the human race

Unfortunately, Brahma's sons could not create living beings because they originated from desire, perception and touch. Brahma instructed his son, Daksa Prajapati, the great chief, to worship the goddess Kalika, mother of the universe for assistance. For 3,000 years he practiced penance and sacred rites on the northern shore of the ocean of milk in hopes of seeing the goddess.

Daksa lived on air alone for a long period, then drank only water for a while before living on leaves. Finally, Kalika, in the form of Durga appeared to him while he was practicing the eight restraints of yoga: yama, niyama, asana, pranayama, pratyahara, dharana, dhyana and Samadhi.

The four-armed goddess, seated on a lion, was magnificent. She held a blue lotus in one hand and a sword in another. Durga, giver of creation and the abode of safety, expressed her pleasure with his devotion and told him, "there is nothing which shall not be granted to you." He returned to his hermitage and began the process of creation by the power of his mind.

For all of his effort, Daksa did not produce the desired results. Although he worked at it for a long time, his creations remained stationary and lifeless. At a loss for what to do he informed his father, Brahma, the Creator, that his creations were not flourishing.

Daksa's children

Upon hearing the news, Brahma suggested that Daksa take Virini, the beautiful daughter of Virana, lord of the five tribes, as a consort to create subjects.

Heeding his advice, Daksa married Virini and fathered 5,000 children, known as the Haryasvas, to populate the earth. Seeing Daksa's great progress Narana, the sage, suggested his sons explore the universe before setting themselves to the task of their own creations. They followed his advice and explored the depths of the universe, ultimately, getting lost, never to be seen in their homeland again.

Daksa Prajapati, devastated over the loss of his Haryasvas sons, then fathered 1,000 Brahmanas sons, known as the Saval. When they were ready to carry on with the work of creation, Narada suggested they first explore the universe and try to find their lost brothers. Taking his advice, the Saval sons ventured out and found some of their lost brothers but ended up just as lost, never to find their way home.

Mourning the loss of his second set of sons, Daksa fathered 60 daughters with Panchajani, daughter of Virani. He gave 10 to Dharma who became the mothers of the gods (Devas). The other 50 mothered all of the other beings in the universe with five celestial bodies, including Chandrana, the moon.

Vishnu's ten incarnations

According to the *Matsyamahapurana*, the present world cycle is the seventh, known as Vaivasvata. In this cycle Vishnu incarnates into 10 different forms to protect the world from evil. His incarnations follow an evolutionary pattern, from fish to reptile, to animals, to man and, finally, the destroyer and creator, Kalkin.

1. Matsya: Vishnu as the fish

Toward the end of the sixth world cycle in the present day of Brahma, King Caksusa Manu gave his kingdom to his son, Vaivasvata. One day while the new king was practicing libation of water to the names of his ancestors a small fish came into his hands along with the water. The merciful and compassionate king placed it in his jar of water. Within a day the fish outgrew the jar and the king placed him in a pitcher that he outgrew in less than a day. The fish cried for mercy and begged to be rescued so the king placed him in a well that he soon outgrew. He was relocated to a tank of water that he outgrew in a day. When he outgrew his next home in the Ganges the king set him free in the ocean where he continued to grow until he nearly filled the entire sea.

The king proclaimed great respect for the fish who revealed himself as Matsya, the first incarnation of Vishnu. He told King Vaivasvata there would come a day in the near future when rain would stop for 100 years and the universe would suffer a dire famine. All the inferior beings in the universe would be scorched to death by the seven ordinary rays of the sun that would eventually become seven times more powerful. Sesa, the thousand-hooded serpent upon which the universe rests, will shoot out from his abode in the lower regions, sending out venomous flames from his 1,000 mouths and Siva's third eye will open, reducing heaven, earth and hell to ashes with a furious fire. Afterward seven destructive clouds will rise from the vapors created by the heat of Sivas third eye, the Sun and Sesa, causing torrential rain that will devour the earth.

Matsya instructed the king to accept a boat that would be presented to him by the Devas (gods) before the deluge and bring on board the seed of creation and the sacred *Vedas*. Afterward, he was to fasten the boat to Matsya's horn using Sesa, the serpent, as a rope.

According to Matsya, the only things exempt from the destruction beside himself would be the moon, the sun, Vishnu, Brahma, the sacred river, Marmada, the great sage, Markandeya, the sacred *Vedas*, the *Puranas*, Shiva and the sciences. This partial dissolution would be the end of the reign of King Caksuka Manu in the sixth world cycle giving way to the next world cycle.

At the beginning of the dissolution King Vaivasvata Manu used his yogic powers to gather a pair of each living being onto the boat. After securing it to Matsya's horn he saluted the Lord, got on board and was taken to a safe place to wait for the dissolution to take place.

2. Koorma: Vishnu as the tortoise

During the partial dissolution the demons (asuras) were getting increasingly stronger than the gods. Fearful of being overpowered, the gods called upon Vishnu for help. He proposed churning the ocean of milk to get the nectar of immortality (amrita) so the gods would have the power to become invincible. They used the mountain, Mandara, to churn the ocean. To prevent it from sinking to the bottom Vishnu incarnated into Koorma and supported the mountain on his back. The gods ate the nectar of immortality as it floated to the surface of the ocean and became invincible.

3. Varah: Vishnu as the boar

During the great flood a demon named Hiranyaksha abducted Prithivi, goddess of the earth, taking her to the bottom of the cosmic ocean. Vishnu, incarnated as Varah and rescued her after a long battle with the demon on the ocean floor. He carried the beautiful goddess carefully on his tusks to the surface of the ocean. As they approached, continents, mountains and rivers manifested, creating the ideal place for Vaivasvata Manu to dock his boat.

4. Narasimha, Vishnu as the man/lion

In Vishnu's absence a gatekeeper to his heaven named Hiranyakasipu performed some evil deeds and was condemned to live the rest of his life as a demon. He did penance in the name of Brahma who eventually granted him special powers that protected him from harm by humans, animals or weapons, making him invincible.

These new powers gave the demon confidence to wage war against the gods, making their lives difficult. When he and his army began winning battles the gods complained to Vishnu who incarnated as Narasimha, a half man, half lion. He hid behind a pillar in front of the demon's house, grabbing him in the doorway, overpowering his blessings and mauling him to death with his sharp claws. The gods, pleased with his demise, resumed their peaceful lives.

5. Vamana: Vishnu as a dwarf

Through penance, Bali, the grandson of Hiranyakasipu, became extremely powerful and set himself on a course to rule the three worlds, heaven, earth and hell. His first order of business was to avenge his grandfather, so with great anger he expelled the gods from heaven. In desperation the gods called out for help from Vishnu once again.

Vishnu presented himself to the demon as Vamana, a dwarf, requesting a place to meditate that he could encircle with only three steps. Bali granted the request in hopes the gesture would generate good fortune. Instead, Vamana took advantage of the situation, transforming into Trivikrama, the giant. With his first step he encircled the heavens, with his second the earth and as a gesture of kindness for the demons he left the underworld, or hell, to Bali.

6. Parashurama: Vishnu as a human being

Vaivasvata Manu was the first king of the solar dynasty. The people who originated from him established the great Hindu civilization. They adopted the practicalities found in the Dharma (virtue) and created a system of four social classes, (1) Brahmana or Brahmin (priest), (2) Kshatryas (warrior), (3) Vaishya (merchant) and (4) Sudra (servant).

After living in harmony for a long time a rivalry erupted between the Brahmins and the Kshatryas. The misunderstanding was over who guarded the sacred knowledge based on the Vedanta and Yoga. Traditionally, the Brahmins were custodians of the great knowledge although the Kshatryas played an important role in its development. The outcome of the rivalry was war. On the side of the Brahmins, Vishnu, in the form of Parashurama, led the war against the Kshatryas. After 21 battles the Brahmins declared victory and the right to remain custodians of the sacred knowledge. Vishnu sent Kashyapa, teacher of Vedanta and master of Ayur-veda, to propagate the Vedanta philosophy and Ayur-veda around the world. Having fulfilled his mission, Vishnu left for the mountain, Mahendra, to meditate on the Sat-Brahman.

7. Rama: Vishnu as a king

After a long meditation on the mountain, Mahendra, Vishnu divided himself into four parts to be born as the four sons of King Dasharatha; Rama, Bharata, Lakshmana and Shatrughna. One day while his brothers were away the king offered his kingdom to Rama, his favorite son. Upon seeing his brothers were not around and his father's consort was unhappy with the idea, Rama renounced the kingdom and went into voluntary exile, taking Sita, his soul mate, and his brother, Lakshmana, with him. They retreated to the forest where Rama fought many battles against powerful monsters trying to seduce Sita. One day Ravana, the evil king of (Sri) Lanka abducted Sita and brought her to his capital where he kept her in a garden of Ashoka trees.

The king of birds was mortally wounded by the evil ruler when he tried to prevent the abduction but managed to alert Rama and his brother before dying. They performed the last rites on his remains and headed south to rescue Sita.

They first entered the land of the monkeys and had a friendly duel with Sagria, brother of the monkey king. Then Rama killed the monkey king, winning sovereignty over the monkey land. He appointed Jugriva, one of his generals, to rule and commissioned the leaders of the monkey army to search for Sita. Hanuman, one of the generals, searched the southern forest and found Shampati, a sage, who provided information leading him to the goddess.

Sita was guarded by female monsters pressing her to 'share the bed' with Ravana when Rama and his monkey army arrived, destroying the city and killing many. Rama killed Ravana with one arrow and freed Sita who ascended in the car with him. Feeling victorious, Hanuman and his army followed them back to their kingdom where Rama reigned for many years.

8. Krishna: Vishnu as a sage

In the *Vayaviyasamhita*, after Vishnu incarnated as Krishna, Upamanyu (Shiva) instructed him in the philosophy of yoga. He learned the meaning and goal of yoga for the Vaivasvata world cycle.

Yoga in the Upamanyu tradition:

- Mantrayoga: concentration on mantra
- Sparsayoga: pranayama with mantra
- Bhavayoga: meditation on the universe
- Mahayoga: meditation on Shiva

Mahayoga is based on the eight restraints: yama, niyama, asana, pranayama, pratyahara, dharana, dhyana and samadhi.

1. Yama: restrain from violence, theft, sex and greed.
2. Niyama: positive state of being; pure, content, attentive, repentant and japa (recitation).
3. Asanas: originally eight types; svastika, padma, ardhendu, vira, yoga, prasadhita, paryanka, yathesta.
4. Pranayama: control of the breath.
5. Pratyahara: withdrawal of the senses.
6. Dharana: concentration within
7. Dhyana: contemplation on Siva/Sakti, the universal-self.
8. Samadhi: enlightenment, the soul (Atman) merges with Shiva.

9. Gautama Buddha, Vishnu as Siddartha

Siddartha was a prince, born around the middle of the sixth century B.C. in Padeira, in the northern district of Gorakpur, India. He lost his mother seven days after his birth, and at 16, married his cousin, Yasodhara. They lived with their son, Rahula, in the confines of his palace for many years enjoying the privileges and pleasures of royal life.

As the years went by Siddartha became aware of the sorrow and suffering outside of his perfect world. At the age of 29, driven by his desire to understand and relieve the suffering and sorrow of the world, he left his family and retired to the forest to learn from two revered Brahman sages, Arada Kalama and Vdraka Ramaputra. Kamala was a follower of Kapila, founder of the Sankhya sect of philosophy, and a strong believer in the Atman. Ramaputra believed the highest level of spirituality was a state of neither consciousness or unconsciousness.

Dissatisfied with their teachings Siddartha moved on to learn from priests responsible for running temples. He hoped to learn how to escape suffering and sorrow. Instead, he was revolted and dismayed to see animal sacrifices at the alters of the gods. Siddartha had come to believe the only way to practice true religion was to live a moral life. He preached to them that destroying life to make amends for evil deeds was useless, but they did not listen.

Disappointed, Siddartha left the temples and found a group of Udraka students practicing austerities. With admiration for their enthusiasm and determination, Siddartha joined them.

A few years of the austere life caused Siddartha's body to become extremely weak. After bathing in the Nairanjana River one day he struggled to get out, staggered and fell to the ground. He lay there for some time before Sujata, the oldest daughter of a herdsman, found him near death, took him home and nursed him back to health. Siddartha concluded that the ascetic way was not going to help him end suffering and sorrow and gave it up.

Then, one day while meditating under a fig tree, he had a powerful insight and, suddenly, understood all that was wrong with the spiritual disciplines of his time. He realized that suffering and sorrow originated from selfish actions and developed the Ten Perfections to help escape these human conditions:

1. Paramudita: generosity
2. Vamala: physical and mental purity
3. Prabhakari: humility
4. Archismati: chastity
5. Sudurjaya: self-mastery
6. Abhimukhi: wisdom
7. Durangama: detachment
8. Acala: submission
9. Sadhumati: Samadhi
10. Dharmamegha: one with the universe/ Sat-Brahman

10. Kalkin: the last incarnation of Vishnu

The final incarnation of Vishnu is expected to appear at the end of the present world cycle, setting off the beginning of the next partial dissolution that will cleanse the world with scorching heat and torrential rains. As we approach the end of Vaivasvata Manu, the current world cycle, it is written that humanity will face a breakdown of civilization and a loss of spiritual and moral values. Kalkin will prepare and save the seed of civilization, the *Vedas*, the *Puranas* and all the other works of importance to civilization for Savani Manu, the next world cycle.

Sages

Maharishi Patanjali

"O Brahmana! I am Narayana, I am the creator and destroyer of all. I am known as Ananta and Sesa."
Sri-Bhagavana

According to the myth, Ananta reincarnated as Maharishi Patanjali, divine lord of serpents, teacher of Samkhya and codifier of yoga in the most comprehensive work ever compiled.

Patanjali's *Sutras* are easy to learn, follow and practice, even for beginners on the path. The system is intended to abolish hindrances (mental hang-ups) and Karma that prevent us from making progress in the study and development of the self.

Patanjali described yoga as concentration, as does the *Sivapurana*. A commentary about the sutras by James H. Woods in his *Harvard University Oriental Series, Volume 17*, defines yoga as 'concentration to restrict fluctuations of the mind' based on the stem word 'yuj-a' indicating concentration rather than the stem word 'yuj-i' indicating conjunction or union.

Patanjali's *Yoga Sutras* laid out standards and guidelines for the ideal practice of Raja Yoga and self-cultivation in four volumes; (1) concentration, (2) means of attainment, (3) supernormal powers and (3) isolation.

1. Concentration

Concentration (yoga) is the focus of the first volume. It outlines methods to develop the power of concentration, defined as restriction of the mind (citta), or the three elements of thought, known as gunas, that also represent the principal building blocks of nature: brightness - sattva, activity - rajas and inertia - tamas.

Yoga, as concentration, is established after a long period of uninterrupted practice. It requires determination and focused attention, which is essential throughout the stages of mental development:

- Restlessness (ksipta): symptoms include thirst, passion, violence, lust, jealousy and desire.
- Infatuation (mudha): darkness and ignorance from lack of spirituality, sloth and too much sleep.
- Distraction (viksipta): instability generated by natural causes, disease or lack of vitality.
- Single-intent (ekagra): focus comes clear, hindrances dwindle and bonds of karma loosen.
- Restricted (niruddha): the soul takes control of the mind through the power of yoga (concentration)

Breath control also cultivates stillness of the mind and concentration. It is important to learn healthy breathing for daily health and essential to learn proper breath control as part of your yoga practice.

According to ancient texts, the self is nothing more than an atom in darkness that becomes conscious by pondering upon itself, consciously saying, "I am", expressed by the mystic syllable "OM".

The transcendental-self evolves from brightness and resides in the 12-petal lotus of the heart. Faith or belief in the transcendental-self (Ishvara) is the foundation for concentration.

2. Means of Attainment

Patanjali's second volume explains yoga of action in four divisions. The goal is to focus the mind on the transcendental-self to manifest a state of vividness.

1. Self-castigation
2. Mantra, repetition of mystic syllables
3. Study of texts on liberation.
4. Devotion to the transcendental-self.

Included in the Means of Attainment are five hindrances to avoid or overcome:

1. Undifferentiated-consciousness: mental impressions that prevent the mind from understanding the self.
2. Feeling-of-personality: generated by seeing through the self.
3 Passion: usually based on greed, thirst and desire for power and pleasure.

Origins

4. Aversion: lack of will power to overcome pain, repulsion and anger, the cause of most human afflictions.
5. Will-to-live: generated from spiritual ignorance, one wrongly identifies the body as the main being and becomes driven by instinct to survive.

Karma is rooted in the hindrances and affects us whether we know it or not. The result is extreme anguish or pure joy, depending on the intention of our actions. Regular practice has the potential to cultivate concentration and diminish the five hindrances to reverse the cycle of karma and reach a state of self-mastery.

To assist the practitioner on the path, Patanjali codified the two restraints, or moral codes of behavior, and six angas, or limbs. Taken from Krisna's Maha Yoga, they comprise the eight-fold path.

Restraints - Moral Codes of Behavior

1. Yama: five abstentions.
"Thou shall not harm, lie, steal, be sensual or greedy."
2. Niyama: five observances
"Thou shall be clean, content, self-controlled, studious and devoted to the transcendental-self (Ishvara)."

According to Patanjali, following these virtues of moral behavior could generate positive effects such as absence of danger, effective speech, the arrival of unsought wealth, vigor of body and mind, steadiness of attention, control of the senses, great happiness, perfection of body, intuition and realization of one's true self.

Angas: External Limbs

1. Asana: balanced posture to prevent physical obstacles during meditation. Once mastered, the foundation for real yoga (concentration) has been established.
2. Pranayama: breath control
3. Pratyahara: withdrawal of the senses from the outer world to focus on the transcendental-self

Angas: Internal Limbs

1. Dharana: concentration
2. Dhyana: meditation
3. Samadhi: contemplation and self-realization

3. Supernormal Powers

Supernormal powers come from practicing constraints based on fixed attention, or uninterrupted thought. Patanjali suggests focusing on the navel, heart-lotus, light within the mind, the tip of the nose or tongue, or any external object or place on the body. The mind empties itself to become one with the point of focus.

Although supernormal powers develop as a result of practice, the ultimate goal is to develop the eight perfections:

1. Atomization: mastery of the atoms of the body.
2. Levitation: mastery of body's density/weight.
3. Magnification: ability to expand the body to a massive size.
4. Extension: ability to touch the moon with the fingertips.
5. Efficacy: ability to dive into and emerge from earth as if in water.

6. Mastery: power to subjugate the elements.
7. Sovereignty: power to produce, absorb and arrange the elements.
8. Will: power to subjugate time, space and matter.

Mastery of the eight perfections gives the yogi full power over all states of existence, a level of purity that leads to Isolation.

4. Isolation

Methods used by yogis to reach a state of Isolation include concentration, castigation, spells and drugs. Karma and hindrances are destroyed and the path to liberation is cleared.

Six Limb Path

"They name posture, breath, restraint, (prana-samrodha), sense withdrawal, concentration, meditation and ecstasy as the six limbs of Yoga."
                                            Goraksha-Paddhati

The *Goraksha-Paddhati*, compiled in the 12th or 13th century AD, and the *Hatha Yoga Pradipika*, (*Light on Yoga*), compiled by Yogi Swatmarama sometime in the 14th century, establish the six limb path of Yoga, beginning with asanas. According to an introduction to a translation of *The Hatha Yoga Pradipika* by Panchan Sinh in 1915, Yogi Swatmarama discards the yamas and the niyamas because they are moral codes of behavior that, he felt, would come naturally as one's practice develops and evolves.

Unlike Buddhist and Jain scriptures, and Pantanjali's *Yoga Sutras*, the *Hatha Yoga Pradipika* does not impose yamas and niyamas (self-control, rules of conduct and observances). Yogi Swatmarama considered them religious rather than spiritual. He was also aware that trying to follow yamas and niyamas created more mental stress than peace of mind.

The *Hatha Yoga Pradipika* advocates discipline and purification of the body through Hatha Yoga. It develops self-discipline, self-control and, ultimately, induces natural spiritual development.

Yogis following the path of physical culture and six limb yoga practiced mainly physical asanas, and practitioners of spiritual culture and the eight limb path chose the more meditative series. Variations and modifications evolved over the centuries as they were passed from teacher to student in the oral tradition.

The two paths within the practice of Yoga are not always clear to western practitioners and is often the cause of confusion. Understanding the differences can help to clarify the goals and direction of your personal practice.

"Individuals who take to the practice of Asanas are of two types: Those who seek only physiological advantages and those who are anxious to secure spiritual advantages also. People of the first type may be called physical culturists, and those of the second type may be termed spiritual culturists."
Popular Yoga Asanas

* * *

*"What is desirable in body culture is the
harmonious development of power
over the voluntary actions of muscles and the
involuntary processes of health, lungs, stomach and,
other organs and important glands.
This is what gives health, and, is the
scientific principle underlying the Yoga exercises."*

Bishnu Ghosh

Yoga Challenge® Lineage

The *Yoga Challenge® I* is a system of classic, beginning Hatha Yoga derived from the 84 classic asanas of the Ghosh/Bikram lineage of physical culturists. This unique sequence of asanas is the foundation of my training and practice.

My teacher, Bikram Choudhury, was trained by Shree Bishnu Charan Ghosh, founder of Ghosh's College of Physical Education, in Calcutta, India (est. 1924). As a young master of yoga, he was sent to Japan and the United States in the early 1970's to establish the Yoga College of India.

Bishnu Ghosh trained at the Ranchi School for Boys, founded in 1917 by his brother, Paramhansa Yogananda, founder of the Self-Realization Fellowship and author of *Autobiography of a Yogi*.

Yogananda's teacher, Sri Yukteswar, author of *The Holy Science*, was a disciple of Lahiri Mahasaya, the first non-sadhu to learn yoga. Babaji Nagaraj, a "sanyasing" or "sadhu" initiated Mahasaya in 1861.

Bishnu, a physical culturist, worked with his friend and colleague, Swami Sivananda Saraswati to develop systems of Hatha Yoga for health and fitness, derived from the 84 classic asanas of this lineage.

Sivananda's teachings originate from Yogi Matsyendranath, regarded as the first human teacher of Hatha Yoga. Matsyendranath's chief disciple, Gorakhnath, was guru to Yogi Swatmarama, author of the *Hatha Yoga Pradipika*.

~ ~ ~

In a commentary to a 1985 translation of the *Hatha Yoga Pradipika*, Swami Muktibodhananda Saraswati explains, *"the main objective of Hatha Yoga is to create an absolute balance of the interacting activities and processes of the physical body, mind and energy. When this balance is created, the impulses generated give a call of awakening to the central force which is responsible for the evolution of human consciousness. If Hatha Yoga is not used for this purpose, its true objective is lost."*

The 84 classic asanas that the *Yoga Challenge*® systems derive from are one of several, passed from teacher to student. It has evolved over the centuries from an original series yet to be identified. It is believed to originate from a system codified around the 10th century AD, by Yogi Matsyendranath, founder of the Nath sect.

SCIENCE

"When posture and form are perfect the movement that follows is perfect as well."
                              Taisen Deshimaru

Science of Yoga

In spite of the mythological foundation of Hatha Yoga, it is technically scientific and medically therapeutic for a wide range of maladies. Clinical studies have been, and continue to be, conducted around the world on the therapeutic benefits of Hatha Yoga for a wide variety of chronic illnesses such as asthma, diabetes, depression and menopause.

Science is knowledge about nature or the universe, based on facts from study, observation and experiments. It is understanding the different forces in nature and how they respond to our actions. For example, if you put too much weight on the outside of your standing foot in the standing bow, you will fall over. Not only is your weight out of center, your muscles are not evenly engaged, creating muscular imbalance

Hatha Yoga is a science developed to keep body and mind healthy and strong. Asanas are designed to be performed with the skeleton in geometric alignment with the earth. Movement, balance and stretching follow the natural laws of physics that apply to everything in nature and the universe.

The science of Hatha Yoga practice is knowledge about the benefits of the asanas and how to practice in balance or harmony with the laws of nature. Therapeutic Hatha Yoga practice is based on the science of anatomy, astronomy, nature, geometry, physics and art/aesthetics.

Science of Practice

Hatha Yoga is a mind/body method of exercise. The foundations of Yoga *Challenge®* practice are concentration, alignment, proper weight distribution, breath control and mindful movements. Each contributes to the optimum development of posture, body and mind.

A useful practice tool for alignment is a plumb line. Make one by attaching a long piece of string to something heavy enough to pull it down in a straight line when hung from above. They are also available in hardware stores. The bob, or weight at the end of the string is pulled down by the earth's gravity. Use the straight line, perpendicular to the earth, created by the string, as the focal point for aligning your body.

The plumb line represents the axis of the body and the line of gravity that passes vertically through it. Most of your body's weight should be centered along this line during practice and, ideally, throughout the day. In a properly aligned body, the center of gravity and center of weight are in front of the first or second segment of the sacrum.

Known as the Central Position, standing in alignment, is used by physical therapists and the entire medical community as the standard for proper posture. The range of motion of major joints in the body are measured from the central position using conceptual lines and planes in relation to the axis, or center, of your body. Understanding this concept will help to improve your personal practice and teachings immensely.

Three planes divide the body into equal halves from the center, or axis: front and back; right and left; top and bottom. Planes are conceptual lines in space that serve as principal tools in the science of body mechanics and alignment.

Conceptual use of the three planes is an essential tool for true alignment and measurement of progress in your yoga practice. The planes are used as the standard to guide you towards the ideal position throughout this manual. Visualize the planes crossing at your center of gravity creating 90° angles. Try to stay within the lines of the planes as you move into, hold and move out of the poses.

Following these lines and planes can help restore faulty alignment and bad posture that can cause chronic pain and, in some instances, physical deformity. A mirror and plumb line are helpful for measuring progress from consistent yoga practice. The ideal alignment may not be attained instantly, however, gradually and progressively, as strength, flexibility, concentration and balance develop, alignment also improves and the asanas become easier.

Begin by comparing the 'ideal posture' of each asana to your actual posture. Note the variables of your personal limitations and modify the posture as suggested. Remember, in most cases, the modifications are temporary, the ideal posture is the goal. Visualize the planes, lines and axis as you move into, hold and move out of the asanas.

". . . the faithful student will find that the yoga exercises invariably and consciously develop his will power along with his bodily strength."
Bishnu Ghosh

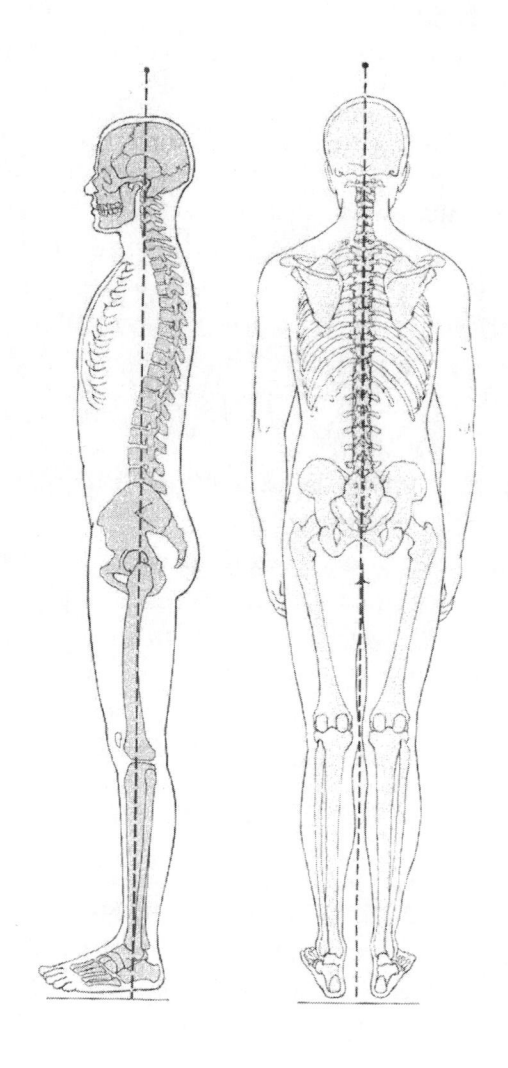

Axis and Planes

The anatomical or central position of the body is an upright and erect posture, perpendicular to the earth. It is measured against a conceptual, perpendicular line, originating from the center of the earth, called the axis. Movement takes place along your axis, which is in alignment with the earth's.

Planes

Sagittal Plane:

The name originates from the sagittal suture of the skull. It divides the body into right and left halves. Movements in the Sagittal plane are to the left and right (abduction and adduction) of the axis without twisting or bending.

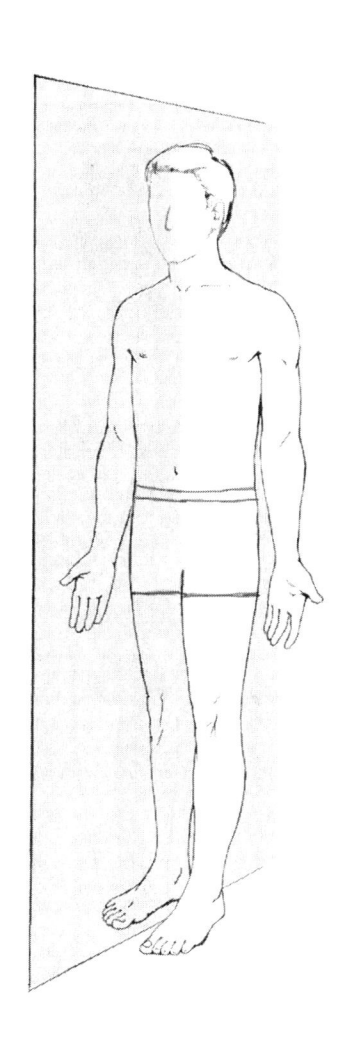

Example: moving in the saggital plane from the central position into the Lateral Half Moon or Triangle, the body only moves from side to side along the lines of this plane.

Science

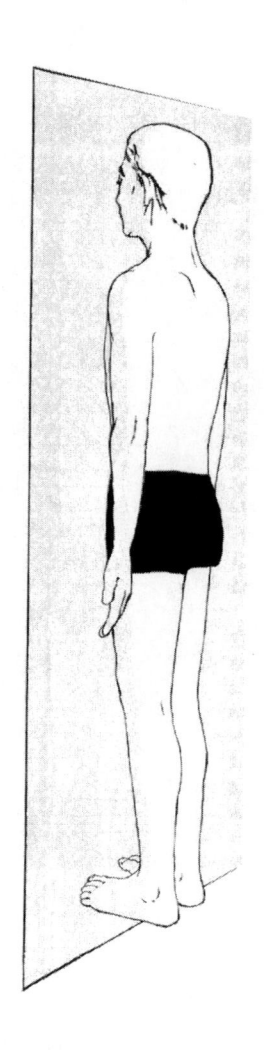

Coronal Plane:

The name originates from the coronal suture of the skull. It divides the body into front and back halves. The movements in this plane are back (extension) and forward (flexion) stretches.

Example: Back-bend and forward-bend in the Half-Moon series.

Transverse Plane:

A horizontal plane, the transverse, divides the body into upper and lower portions. The point at which the three planes intersect in the body is the center of gravity and usually supports most of the body's weight. In an ideal posture the center of gravity is slightly forward of the first or second segment of the sacrum. Movements in the Transverse plane are medial and lateral rotation, and horizontal extension or compression.

Examples: Separate-Leg-Stretching, Head-to-Knee or Spinal Twist

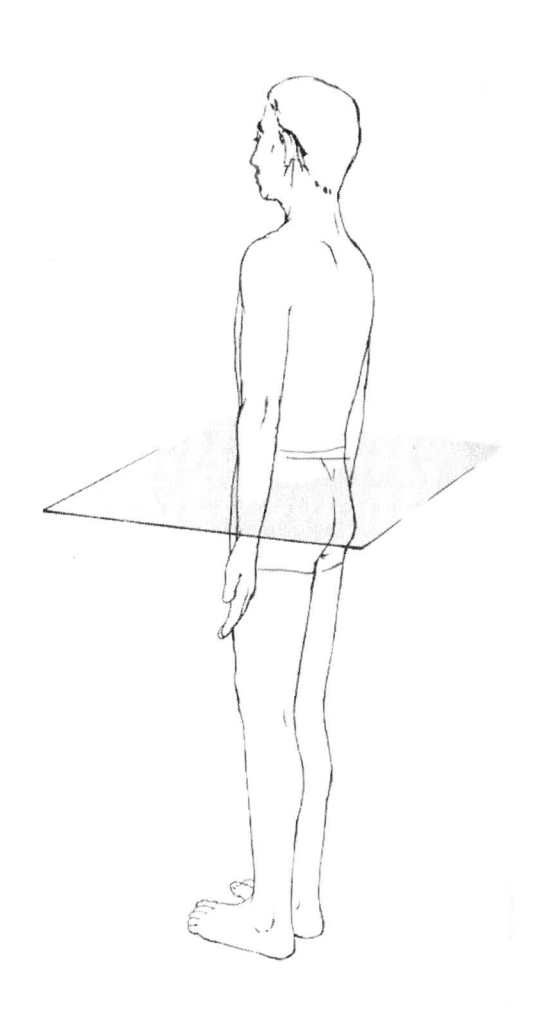

If it seems impossible to align with the planes it only means that you have a goal and a focus. Strive to improve gradually and progressively. Performing the postures perfectly is less important than making a sincere effort. Maintain alignment and push to the best of your ability. It does not take long to see progress with regular practice.

Scientific Stretch

A scientific stretch begins with skeletal alignment and proper weight distribution with both feet or sit-bones firmly on the floor. Maintain both as you slowly and evenly move into the postures, stretching muscles with equal but opposite force from the center of the body out. Always stretch muscles and spine from end-to-end.

For example, in Lateral Half Moon, stretch muscles down from waist to floor, and up from waist to fingertips.

"Postures strengthen and develop will and body – physical and mental development are intertwined."
Bishnu Ghosh

* * *

"The body is literally manufactured and sustained by mind."
Yogananda

Science of the Body

Humans manifested from single-cell organisms over more than three billion years of evolution. We are made up of nearly 60-billion cells working in harmony to create a complex series of systems that perform our necessary functions.

Systems of the Body

1. Respiratory
2. Digestive
3. Cardiovascular
4. Vascular
5. Nervous
6. Locomotive

Respiratory System

The body's main source of energy is oxygen, absorbed through the air we breathe. We require a continuous supply that, if compromised in any way, causes cells to die prematurely. Lack of oxygen can be self-inflicted by activities such as smoking, or by things beyond our control such as illness or trauma.

The lungs are the main organs of respiration and are protected by the rib cage. Air, inhaled through the nose or mouth, passes through the larynx, down the wind pipe and into the lungs. Permeated with fine, elastic fibers, the lungs are capable of expanding to increase air capacity that will increase the flow energy and/or circulation. Through a biochemical process oxygen is extracted from air and metabolized into energy in the bloodstream.

The diaphragm, located beneath the lungs and inter-costal muscles, helps to expel air and carbon dioxide from the lungs. Breathing can be consciously controlled or completely ignored and left to the automatic nervous system run by the brain. Energy manifested by the body from oxygen manages the mechanics of the body, facilitates movement, thoughts and sounds. Breathe consciously for optimum health and fitness.

Digestive System

In addition to oxygen, all the systems, organs and tissue that constitute the body require nutrition to generate the necessary energy to function effectively. The digestive organs absorb nutrients from the food we eat into the digestive system to be broken down and processed into the blood stream for distribution to cells throughout the body.

The digestive system functions semi-automatically, in that we must choose and ingest the nutrients, and we can oversee and control daily elimination of the waste. Proper diet and exercise are the two most natural methods to ensure elimination.

For the yoga practitioner considering a vegetarian diet, the importance of a healthy balance cannot be overstated. Although there are benefits to vegetarian and raw diets, they can also deplete the body of important nutrients needed for optimum health and fitness if not properly balanced. It takes a lot of vegetables and grains to replace nutrients provided in meat, fish or foul. It is important to educate yourself or consult a nutritionist before you begin.

A moderate diet, including small amounts of healthy, uncontaminated fish, poultry and/or meat may be an easier path to follow. A nutritionist can help to develop balanced menus based on your personal lifestyle and nutritional needs.

Cardiovascular System

The cardiovascular system has two main functions. The first is to distribute nutrients, oxygen and hormones throughout the body, and the second is to remove metabolic waste. The heart, an organ and a muscle the size of a fist, is the main force behind this process. Located behind the sternum, the heart pumps blood throughout the network of blood vessels covering the entire body. It pumps every minute that we are alive whether we think about it or not.

According to clinical studies, the heart of a sedentary person beats an average of around 100,000 times in a day. Basically, it is the minimum number necessary for the body to maintain itself with minimum energy and movement. Minimum maintenance, however, usually leads to major health problems in later years.

Unlike breath control, increasing our daily number of heartbeats can only be achieved with movement or exercise that requires energy, thereby forcing the heart to pump faster. This not only increases circulation to produce energy needed to move and exercise, it strengthens and nourishes the heart.

Vascular System

The vascular system is a dense network of vessels that transports blood to every part of the body. The main arteries spread away from the heart, passing into the organs and tissues where they form an intricate system of very small hair-like vessels called capillaries. Blood circulates through the capillaries, releasing nutrients, oxygen and other substances into cells while absorbing waste products for removal.

Capillaries feed the depleted blood into larger veins that transport it back to the right side of the heart. It is then pumped into the lungs where it expels carbon dioxide and absorbs oxygen before returning to the left side of the heart to be pumped into the circulatory system once again.

Nervous System

A fine network of fibers throughout the body makes up the nervous system. It monitors and regulates all the functions of the body by sending tiny electrical signals of information from one part of the body to another. The nerves grow out from the brain and spinal cord, branching out, with very fine nerve endings, to every part of the body. Most nerves are in bundles, like ropes, forming thick strands, with the thickest of all being the sciatic nerve, that runs down both legs.

The brain controls our thinking process and nearly all of the body's functions and movements. It also processes sensory impressions that manifest feelings, memory and speech. The cerebrum, seat of consciousness and higher mental functions, such as thinking, reasoning, emotions and memory, occupies most of the cranial cavity. The brain stem and cerebellum, located under the cerebrum, control basic functions of the body such as coordination of movements and visual and auditory sensations.

A mature brain weighs approximately 2.5 pounds, and requires 20% of the blood supply. Regular, consistent yoga practice stimulates circulation and cleansing of the blood which contributes to the long-term health of your brain.

Locomotive System

Bones, joints and muscles make up the locomotive system. They create the internal framework, or skeleton of the body with more than 200 bones and 100 joints. It protects the organs and produces corpuscles (red and white blood cells) in the marrow. The skeleton is surprisingly light but has an enormous capacity to withstand stress.

Joints of the skeleton, linked to bone by cartilage, facilitate movement, with the shape of the joint dictating the movements allowed. Major joints include: hinge, saddle, ball and socket, and pivot, or rotational. Ligaments stabilize the joints and prevent bones from being pulled apart by movement.

More than 600 voluntary skeletal muscles, attached to the skeleton, provide stability, support and, the ability to move limbs and perform voluntary movements. Keeping the body upright is among the unique functions these muscles perform.

Movements of the body are facilitated by different muscle groups that work in opposite pairs, whether you are lifting an arm or walking across the room. Muscles contracting in the same direction are called synergists and those pulling in opposite directions are called antagonists.

Smooth muscles are categorized as involuntary muscles and cannot be controlled by the human consciousness. The fibers of these muscles create the walls of the blood vessels, stomach and intestines. Cardiovascular muscles are also involuntary.

Science

" Yoga is of very little use, if studied theoretically."
Pancham Sinh

PRACTICE

Mind/Body Practice

Practice is the only way to develop concentration, build muscles, improve alignment, increase energy and reduce stress all at the same time. To begin, get familiar with the *Yoga Challenge® I* system and your body. Observe your limitations and level of proficiency, and work accordingly. Distinguish the difference between pains from stretching muscles and pain that indicates injury.

Be patient and consistent. Do not push yourself when there is pain from strain, and do not sacrifice alignment to advance into a posture. Yoga postures improve naturally as muscle strength, balance and flexibility develop. Mindful, regulated breath and relaxation are essential, but usually the last and most difficult to master.

Timing

The *Yoga Challenge® I* is a one-hour series. In a studio, where timing is essential, spend 1 to 1.5 minutes on each posture, holding for 10 seconds. If you have the time and inclination, feel free to move more slowly or hold the postures longer.

1. Begin every posture with mindful, regulated breath and continue throughout the exercise.
2. Balance and align the body before moving into a posture for proper muscle and skeletal development.
3. Observe and maintain alignment, form and weight distribution throughout the pose.
4. Once 'in' the pose, release tensions with each exhalation and relax further into the stretch.
Note: physical tension must be mentally released to feel physical relief.

5. Refine alignment, balance, form and weight distribution. Reverse movements to return to a central position. Release all tension. Feel breath, circulation and heart rate return to normal.

Alignment & Balance

The body is in 'alignment and balance' with the earth and its gravitational force. Body weight is actually the amount of gravity from the earth pulling the body downward. When our weight is evenly distributed and the skeleton is in alignment with the earth's gravitational force we encounter the least amount of resistance. Therefore, muscles expend less energy to move and balance requires less effort. Stretching muscles in opposite directions with equal strength from your center creates equal, but opposing forces that brings balance.

To balance in a yoga posture align your skeleton and distribute weight evenly between areas of the body on the floor, unless otherwise instructed. Keep your center of weight and center of gravity together. Move slowly into every posture to maintain balance and alignment. Stretch as far as possible from your center without straining or moving out of alignment. This method will properly develop muscles and prevent injury. Balance develops and becomes effortless when
(1) you have plenty of oxygen from proper breathing,
(2) muscles are stretched in equal and opposite directions,
and (3) the body is in alignment and weight is evenly distributed.

"Gravity is the guru.
By aligning our bones with gravity,
we discover the natural wisdom of the body."
A. Thusius & J. Couch

Mindful Breathing

Mindful, healthy breathing is an essential part of *Yoga Challenge®* practice. Depth and rate of inhalation vary according to the postures and the practitioner. Try to avoid holding your breath, which sometimes happens when concentration is focused on other elements of practice. Respiration should be continuous and regulated to provide consistent and sufficient oxygen to the muscles so they can work aerobically and develop properly.

The proper way to exhale is by contracting the diaphragm and abdominal muscles gradually and without strain to expel stagnant air out of the body. This method keeps body and mind healthy and alert. Inhalation through the nose is essential to filter and warm air before it enters the lungs and blood stream. As you breathe in, relax abdominal muscles and feel the lungs expand as they fill with oxygen, pushing the diaphragm downward against the abdominal organs. This pressure helps massage these vital organs to keep them healthy and functioning properly.

Oxygen from breathing is the main source of energy for every function of the body and brain. Nutrients in the food we ingest is our source of fuel. The process of breathing can be managed consciously or automatically by the brain. Beware, adults who leave respiration to the brain may only be getting the minimum amount of oxygen needed to maintain vital bodily functions. It is often not enough oxygen to, among other things, repair damage to the body caused by the rigors of daily life.

> *"Man may exist some time without eating;*
> *a shorter time without drinking;*
> *but without breathing,*
> *his existence may be measured by a few minutes."*
> — Yogi Ramacharaka

Concentration

Hatha yoga requires concentration to manifest the physiological benefits of consistent practice. Consistent, measured breathing, proper alignment, weight distribution and movement within the planes all require concentration. Easy as it sounds, it's actually one of the most difficult elements of practice. Somehow thoughts of the day, past moments or days to come take over. As soon as you find your thoughts have wandered, refocus concentration on your movements, breath or body to continue mindfully. When relaxing, concentrate on your breathing or heartbeat and heart, where the 'self' resides. Exhale tension from every muscle and surrender all your weight and tension to the floor. You must mentally release physical tension to feel physical relief.

Yoga in the Zone

Yoga in the Zone is a moment of perfect equilibrium. Pure science. Energy, strength, form, alignment, movement, balance, breath and timing are in perfect flow with the forces of nature. The body feels weightless and the moment is timeless.

It takes many hours of practice to reach these moments. At the beginning it will be a posture-by-posture experience until the ultimate happens, all the poses in the sequence become connected and effortless. Time and space evaporate.

It all begins with learning the postures and performing them properly.

*"Perfect consciousness is gained through practice.
Death can be evaded of its prey through practice.
And, then let us gird up our loins and,
with a firm resolution, engage in the practice,
having faith, and the success must be ours."*
                                    Pancham Sinh

*" . . . whether young, old or too old, sick or lean,
one who discards laziness,
gets success if he practices Yoga."*
                                     Hatha Yoga Pradipika

Yoga Challenge® Practice

The *Yoga Challenge® I* is an excellent series for general health and fitness that anyone can practice. Modifications were developed to address a variety of limitations and injuries of students who practiced with me over the last 30 years. They are based on knowledge passed to me by my teacher, more than 100,000 hours of personal practice, and countless more teaching, reading and researching.

Each *Yoga Challenge®* system is a complete mind/body workout. It is important to become proficient with *Yoga Challenge® I* before moving on to *Yoga Challenge® II* and beyond. It is the most effective way to benefit and progress with minimum risk of injury.

Regardless of age, physical condition or limitations, everyone can benefit from practicing the *Yoga Challenge® I*. Traditionally, in India, Hatha Yoga was taught to children for physical and mental development, utilized by adults for therapeutic purposes, and practiced regularly by the elderly after retirement for health and fitness.

~ ~ ~

Where, When and How

Affirm your decision to practice at home by preparing a space and setting up a feasible practice schedule. A small space can be made into a very functional practice area. Before you begin clear the space, if necessary, and put everything you will need within reach. While practicing, turn off your phone and anything else that may distract you.

A mirror is helpful for alignment and form, but not essential. They can be found at hardware and furniture stores in every price range.

Internal and External Heat

To keep muscles supple and prevent injury, try to warm your space to at least 80° or 85°. Most hardware stores carry small, energy efficient room heaters that are fairly inexpensive.

Working up a moderate sweat from effort helps to cleanse your system and skin, but excessive sweating is not advised. In addition to a variety of possible health problems manifesting from long-term practice in very high heat, it may be difficult to hold and progress in postures when the skin is too slippery and wet. It may also be more difficult to focus within or on the foundations of practice - alignment, weight distribution, and proper movement - due to external distractions created by the heat, i.e., drinking water, wiping perspiration, and limited oxygen. This, however, is a personal opinion. For those who practice in a hot room, it is important to be aware of the following.

Our bodies maintain a core temperature of 98.6° F (37°C) through a process called thermoregulation. When performing yoga postures, our core temperature rises due to increased blood flow to engaged muscles, generating heat that is released through respiratory passages and the skin in perspiration to vaporize in the air and cool the body down.

When a room is hotter than your core temperature, the body gains heat from the environment, increasing the core temperature. In an outdoor environment where it is naturally hot and humid, the air with slight breezes evaporates sweat and cools the body in a natural process. A humid, hot room prevents evaporation of perspiration so the body will sweat more in an effort to cool down. Excessive sweating can cause dehydration and, eventually, other more serious conditions. Be sure to drink plenty of fluids before, during and after yoga in a hot room.

Heat Cramps

Although not life threatening, heat cramps are painful muscle spasms that can occur during or after intense physical activity. They are usually in the abdomen or the extremities, often caused by lack of fluids and/or electrolytes.

Heat Exhaustion

Symptoms of heat exhaustion include profuse sweating, dizziness and weakness. If you feel any of these symptoms, stop exercising immediately and try to cool the body down. Drink plenty of fluids immediately and continuously until symptoms pass.

Instructors should escort students with heat exhaustion symptoms to a cooler room to rest. Provide wet towels for the forehead, face and body along with drinking water.

Heat stroke

Heat stroke is a serious condition. It occurs when the core temperature reaches 103°+ and the body can no longer dissipate heat. Symptoms include hot, dry skin and increasing body temperature that can reach up to 106° which can cause organ damage or death. Individuals may be disoriented and confused, and in severe cases unconsciousness may occur. Seek medical assistance. Cool the body with ice, cool water, or any other means possible.

~ ~ ~

The American College of Sports Medicine suggests replacing water at the rate you lose it. To be really sure, weigh yourself before and after exercising. If you weigh less afterward, drink more water. If you weigh more, drink less.

However, the Institute of Medicine warns that drinking too much water during exercise can cause gastrointestinal cramping, nausea and decreased performance. This varies with each individual.

A Harvard University study, at the American College of Exercise suggests checking the color of your urine. If it is darker than lemonade drink more water, sipping it, but never drink more than the amount you actually sweat. They suggest drinking plenty of water two hours before exercising.

~ ~ ~

Do not eat at least three hours before practice. Your body will not be able to digest food and perform asanas at the same time without discomfort. If you drink water during practice, keep it at room temperature so it does not shock your system. Too much water hinders your ability to stretch or lie on your abdomen comfortably, so drink sparingly until the session is over. Drink plenty of room temperature water before and after practice to flush out and cleanse your system.

~ ~ ~

During your final relaxation, *savasana*, try an eye pillow or small towel to block out distractions and light, and really let go of the day. If you have problems lying on your back, add a neck pillow, a tightly rolled up hand towel or two tennis balls in a sock. If necessary, slip another tightly rolled towel under your lower back or knees.

~ ~ ~

Set up your bathroom before you begin so you can go in and shower or soak in a tub about 20 minutes after your practice. An Epsom salt bath is an excellent treatment for sore muscles. A steamy, hot shower cleanses the skin. Try relaxing in the tub or showering by candle light, with your favorite music in the background. Let go of everything that is hanging around in your mind.

Basic Practice Guidelines

1. Do not eat at least three (3) hours before practice.
2. Wear comfortable clothes to stretch.
3. Use a mat or towel for the floor exercises.
4. Practice in a warm, quiet room.
5. Practice at least three times per week.
6. Mirrors are optional, but very helpful.

Preparing Body & Mind

Diet, anything we ingest, feeds the body and the mind. A poor diet manifests on and in the body, impairs our mental state and demoralizes the spirit. It is not necessary to become a vegetarian to practice or teach yoga. It is important to maintain a healthy, nutritious diet and not shock the body with radical dietary changes. If you want to change your diet but are not sure how, it is helpful to consult a nutritionist to establish your needs and diet based on personal health and lifestyle. A knowledgeable nutritionist can suggest a variety of foods and menus to fit your needs.

A lifestyle change that includes Hatha Yoga and a nutritious diet improves overall health and fitness. Most people feel and see a difference within weeks.

Wear comfortable clothing appropriate for the environment or season you are practicing in. Make sure you can stretch easily and the fabric is not too thick or bulky. Keep your feet bare.

~ ~ ~

Before you begin read through the instructions and, if available, watch the DVD carefully. Note any postures you will need to modify and study the modifications. Read your notes periodically to refresh your memory, especially if you practice alone. The information becomes meaningful in different ways as the postures and the routine become familiar. What does not make much sense at one point makes perfect sense at another.

Regular practice improves health and fitness, relaxation, spiritual development, pain relief and mental clarity. It is important to focus your attention on alignment, weight distribution, breath control, and movements from beginning to end. Complete focus on the Self throughout practice is a moving mediation. It is difficult to do, but worth the effort.

In India and throughout the Far East, sitting meditation is preceded by two to three years of Hatha Yoga, tai chi or other physical discipline to prepare the body and focus the mind. Sitting in a lotus position before the body is ready distracts the mind with discomfort and defeats the purpose.

Supplementing with Class Practice

Many of my students practice at home and in hotel rooms when they cannot come to class. Others have moved away and practice at home with the *Yoga Challenge® I* DVD and attend classes in local studios when they can.

Even the most disciplined home-based yoga practitioners benefit from an occasional class with an instructor or mentor. We can always learn from a knowledgeable instructor. Although it would be ideal to take an occasional *Yoga Challenge® I* class with an instructor, the foundations of practice should be the same, regardless of the 'style' - alignment, weight distribution, proper breathing and focus.

Group Practice

It is sometimes more productive and fun to practice in a group. A small group of friends can help each other maintain the discipline for regular practice and help with minor corrections and alignment. This does not mean one person takes the responsibility or role of instructor. Each practitioner should invest the same amount of time in studying the instructions and watching the DVD, if available. Each person needs to prepare for practice following the solo practice guidelines.

Ultimately, we are each responsible for knowing and respecting our personal physical limitations. So it is important to understand the details of each yoga posture and any modifications for your situation.

Yoga Teachers' Practice

It is essential for yoga teachers to practice regularly. Regardless of your hectic life, there is no excuse for not practicing. Otherwise, you are just repeating words.

Yoga is a living energy or entity that becomes a part of you through practice. Yoga is like the sparkles in a top that only glitters when it is moving.

Yoga Challenge® I instructors-in-training do not teach the postures until they learn how to perform them, apply them therapeutically and modify them.

A yoga teacher can only be knowledgeable if they continuously practice and learn. There is always something more to learn about yoga, yourself and yoga, your students and yoga. Learn something new everyday.

Practitioner, Teacher & Entrepreneur

A great yoga practitioner is disciplined and grounded, a great yoga teacher is gifted, and a successful business-yogi must be competitive but ethical. It is a difficult task. However, if you hope to support yourself by teaching, you must practice what you teach, teach what you practice and manage the business of it all wisely. It is worth the time and expense to learn basic bookkeeping, small business management and marketing.

Although some people are able to teach without compensation, most yoga teachers must either charge for their services or have a day job. Teaching yoga as a livelihood is a service business like any other. Laws and rules of commerce and business apply for providing your service as an independent contractor, employee and/or studio owner.

Yoga Etiquette

Etiquette is defined in the dictionary as 'rules of conventional conduct for social behavior or professional conduct'. Although the instructor will ultimately be held responsible, proper conduct, ethical behavior and integrity applies to students as well.

Teachers of Hatha Yoga are first and foremost, human beings, just like everyone else. They have good and bad days, along with the usual personal issues and problems. They do not know the answers to everything and they should not be held to higher standards of conduct than the next person. Activities between consenting adults are personal choices however things turn out, so it is important to think seriously before acting.

Instructors need to be cautious about dating students. If things do not work, you or your employer may notice a drop in attendance, regardless of how great an instructor you are. News travels fast in the changing rooms, especially when it's about an instructor and a student. If you have found the love of your life, which does happen, proceed with integrity and dignity. If you are just looking for a good time, you need to look elsewhere. Otherwise, by natural cause and effect, it will only be a matter of time before perceived unethical behavior of any kind affects the heart of your business – attendance and income.

Ethical conduct should be a part of a yoga teacher's life, both personal and business. Rules of ethical behavior beyond the limits of the law are personal beliefs and cannot be applied to others or forced on them. This is simply to say that we should not have unrealistic expectations of others, as an instructor or a student.

Burnout

Burnout is a state of mind that afflicts teachers and practitioners. My experience is it manifests when the mind is stagnant in teaching or practice. The good news is you can get through it, learn to prevent it and grow from it.

Teaching yoga day in and day out can become monotonous and boring until one day you want to run out the door screaming. Take some time out to assess the causes of your burnout and make positive changes. Begin a new practice schedule, attend a workshop, read something new about yoga or review and enhance your method of practice and/or teaching.

Practice the *Yoga Challenge® I* for long-term health and fitness. If practice begins to feel monotonous focus on different aspects of the series or your practice. For example, focus on breathing, the benefits of each posture, alignment, or the internal organs being stimulated. Throughout an entire session concentrate on the muscles engaged, the spine or weight distribution. If you wander away from practice for a while know that you can always come back to it, no matter what age, whatever your condition.

Keep your mind fresh, maintain a competitive business edge and prevent burnout by tailoring your classes for a specific group you are already familiar with such as, golfers, tennis players, dentists, dancers, etc. Research the chronic problems associated with an activity or career and focus on the benefits of yoga for your chosen group.

Mindful Practice

1. Read through the *Yoga Challenge® I* practice instructions and note any modifications needed and how to do them. If you have any health problems that may be aggravated by physical movements in any part of the system consult your medical practitioner before proceeding.

2. Learn the foundations of practice.

3. For the first few *Yoga Challenge® I* sessions focus on the postures and how to do them. Follow instructions carefully to prevent injury.

4. When you feel comfortable with the postures begin to focus more on the foundations and consciously incorporate them into your practice. Begin with focus on alignment, proper weight distribution and mindful movement.

5. Learn the planes and how to apply them to your practice. Feel your center of weight and how it moves. When performing the postures in alignment with weight evenly distributed you may find your body is not naturally in alignment and it does not stretch as far or balance as well when it is. To develop muscles evenly, do not stretch out of alignment.

6. Regulated, mindful breathing is an essential element of Hatha Yoga practice, however, it is difficult to master because we usually breathe on automatic pilot. It is easier to contemplate and take control of your breathing after you learn the basics of physical practice. When you are comfortable with the flow of the exercises and how to perform them, begin to focus on breathing.

7. While working on your physical practice, broaden your knowledge and understanding of Hatha Yoga by reading. Learn about the origins and history of this ancient practice with classics like the *Vedas*, Patanjali's *Sutras* or something contemporary. This will add to the richness of practice and your appreciation for it.

8. Practitioners: If you have a specific condition such as lower back pain, PMS/menopause, stress, arthritis, etc., do some research on yoga for your condition so you know where to focus your energy. Find an instructor knowledgeable about your condition so they can give you guidance.

    Instructors: Note your own improvements to share with your students. Practice at least five times per week.

Yoga Challenge® I
Asanas

Yoga Challenge® I

*"The primary objective of Hatha Yoga is to control the life force -
for health and mental clarity."*
Yoga Encyclopedia

SERIES

The *Yoga Challenge® I* consists of nine series of asanas and two breathing exercises. It provides a total, comprehensive workout from bones to skin, including internal organs, muscles and the skeletal system. Ideally, the series should be practiced as one continuous exercise, modified to suit the needs of the individual practitioner. Each series develops and stimulates specific areas of the body in a unique way and, together they contribute to the strength and flexibility of the spine.

1. Breathing Series (part 1 & 2)
2. Half Moon Series
3. Awkward Series
4. Transition Series
5. Cobra Series
6. Tortoise Series
7. Stretching Series
8. Abdominal Series
9. Double-Sided Series

STANDING POSTURES

The standing poses are warm-up asanas. They develop strength, flexibility and balance, concentration, will power and patience.

The systematic order of the postures warm-up the joints and muscles in a gradual manner to prevent injuries and enhance the body's potential.

The most effective way to become proficient in the poses is with regular practice, following the instructions carefully. The goal is to stay in alignment with the earth and gravity throughout the session. It should not take more than a few weeks before you can see real progress.

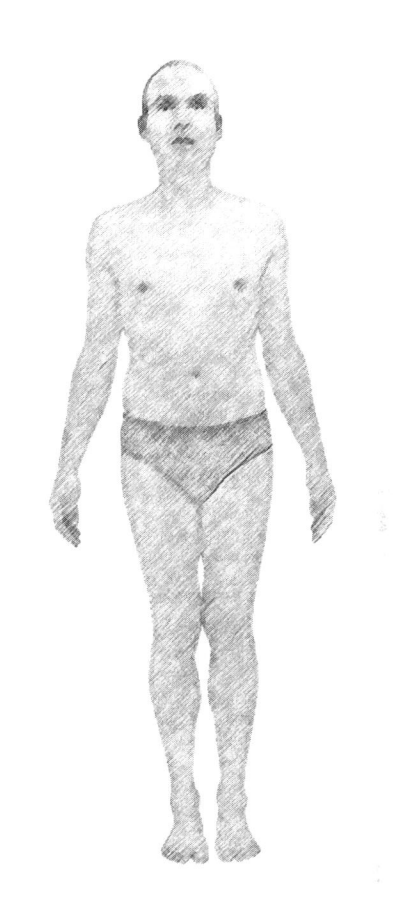

Begin and end all standing postures in the Central Position. Breathing mindfully, stand tall, but relaxed, with arms down, legs, spine, neck and head straight. Hips and shoulders are parallel to the floor and each other, with feet slightly apart and flat on the floor. Weight is evenly distributed between the balls of your feet, toes and heels.

Practice

FLOOR POSTURES

The floor poses are therapeutic, improving the physiological balance of the systems and vital organs. This harmonious balance generates physical health and vitality. The postures also work on the spinal column to stimulate the central nervous system, the brain and all its components for improved concentration and, eventually, interaction with the Self. The best way to master these poses is by following the steps carefully. Know your strengths and weaknesses so you can practice to the best of your ability without strain or injury.

* * *

Instructions incorporate the use of the axis and planes in reference to movements of the body, divided into six even segments: front and back, right and left, bottom and top. Learn and practice yoga using this simple and basic concept of movement in accordance with the laws of nature to master the postures safely and effectively.

STANDING ASANAS
(warm-up postures)

*"The yogi who attempts to practice
without controlling the breath
is compared to a person who wants to
cross the ocean in an unbaked earthen vessel,
which only invites trouble."*
                                         Yoga Encyclopedia

BREATHING SERIES
(part I)

Standing Deep Breathing

Standing deep breathing is a warm-up exercise that prepares the body for practice. It supplies oxygenated blood throughout the body and generates energy to prevent early fatigue which would hinder progress in the postures. At the same time, this exercise expels toxins and waste from the various systems.

Measure progress in this exercise by noting increased air intake when you inhale and by the degree of relaxation you command during the process. Gradually, increase the abdominal pressure applied during exhalation to expel air in the lower lungs.

Center the body on its own axis. Move your head forward and back along the sagittal plane. Use the coronal plane to measure flexibility of neck and arms. Pay attention to the movements of your respiratory muscles, particularly the diaphragm, intercostals and abdominals.

Inhale through your nose, feeling the air flow down the back of the throat into the lungs, expanding them to their fullest capacity, which increases with regular practice. Exhale through the mouth with a slow and steady flow of air, controlled by contracting the abdominal muscles to push and expand the diaphragm against the lungs, forcing air out.

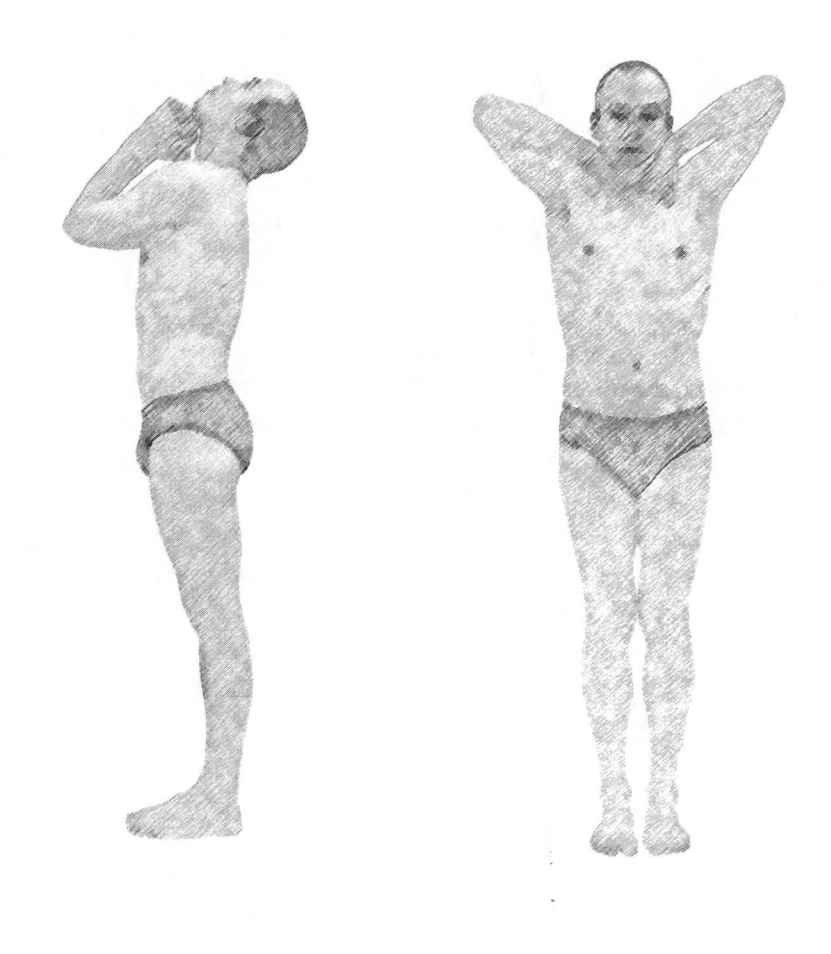

STANDING DEEP BREATHING

1. STANDING DEEP BREATHING
Technique

1. From the Central Position, bring feet together. Interlace fingers under chin, palms and elbows together. Hold leg muscles slightly firm, with spine and legs straight, shoulders and hips square and parallel to floor.

2. Relax head back, chin away from chest. Inhale slowly and steadily through the nose, pressing chin down against interlaced fingers, toward chest, simultaneously raising elbows towards ears.

3. Inhale to a count of six, synchronized with movements of head and elbows. You may have to work on this for a short while before you can do it well. Focus on the air as it passes through the nose, down the back of the throat, filling the lungs, expanding abdominal muscles.

   Inhale as much air as possible without strain, pause one second, then slowly push head back with interlaced fingers, contracting abdominal muscles to press diaphragm against lungs, forcing air out through the mouth. At the same time, bring elbows and wrists together and forward, away from chest, relaxing head back without turning, twisting or straining neck. Align with sagittal plane. Exhale to the same count as the inhale.

4. Repeat 10 times. Relax five seconds in Central Position. *Repeat cycle.* Return to Central Position.

HALF MOON SERIES

Lateral Half Moon, Back Bend, Hands to Feet, Triangle, Standing Separate Leg Head-to-Knee

The poses in the Half-Moon series stretch, compress and twist the spine, abdominal and back muscles progressively and systematically. They also improve flexibility in the legs and, lubricate and limber most of the joints and muscles in the body, improving circulation and general range-of-motion. Most importantly, this series stimulates and strengthens the core of the body and the central nervous system.

Even if you can only stretch a few inches, respect your degree of flexibility and resist any temptation to force or strain. Trust your judgement and allow mind and body to work together. It will always be easier to stretch one side of the body than the other so you must accept that and work with it. Apply extra effort to the stiffer side without straining or compromising alignment or weight distribution. For best results, stay in line with the planes when you stretch.

Breath is regulated according to each asana in the Half-Moon series. For example, when stretching to the side, breathe normally, when stretching back, take shallow, quicker breaths and, when stretching forward, breathe deeply and slowly.

The Half Moon Series disciplines the mind by improving concentration and will power, and enhances the body by improving strength, flexibility and balance. Concentrate on regulating your breath and performing the postures properly and in alignment.

Each pose works on a specific part of the body with specific benefits, from improving flexibility, to building strength and restoring damaged tissue in the body. Pay close attention to the areas in the body being exercised. Identify the muscles you are relaxing, contracting or twisting during the posture to understand your strengths and weaknesses. This will help you to modify or intensify the postures according to your personal needs.

Practice mindfully and feel your body respond to the poses. Proper alignment is essential for the muscles to work and develop simultaneously. Improper alignment and/or weight distribution will strain some muscles and leave others idle. When muscles are out of balance they contribute to the development of poor posture which in many cases is the cause of muscular and joint pains suffered by many. Stretch your muscles rather than bend the body. Keep both feet firmly on the floor with weight evenly distributed.

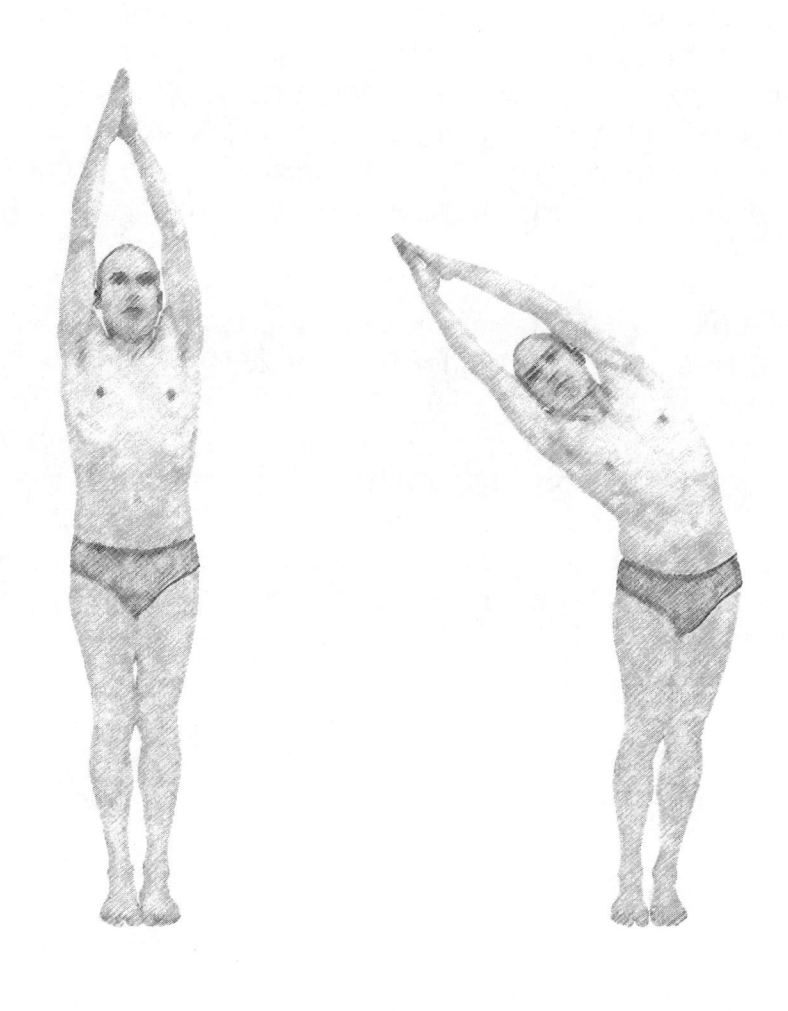

LATERAL HALF MOON

2. LATERAL HALF MOON
Technique

1. From Central Position, with feet together, bring arms over head, palms together, thumbs crossed firmly. Or, interlace three fingers, index fingers and thumbs straight and together. Stretch toward ceiling with chin tucked slightly in, head centered with shoulders and arms. Align ankles, knees, hips, shoulders and head with plumb line or body axis. Maintain alignment throughout posture. Focus on one point in front. Breathe normally.

2. Stretch torso and arms to right following coronal plane. Counterbalance weight by pushing hips slightly left without twisting or turning. Keep hips, abdomen, chest and face forward. If torso droops downward, stretch and turn lower shoulder forward slightly. Align shoulders and hips with coronal plane.

   Note: For sensitive backs, separate feet slightly. Place right hand on hip, fingers forward, thumb back. Bring left arm over head, palm up, fingers and thumb together. Turn head to focus on upper hand. Maintain proper alignment with weight distributed evenly between both feet. Slowly stretch to right side.

3. Breathe normally. Focus on foundations of practice. Hold 10 seconds or longer. *Repeat on left side.* Return to Central Position with arms over head to continue.

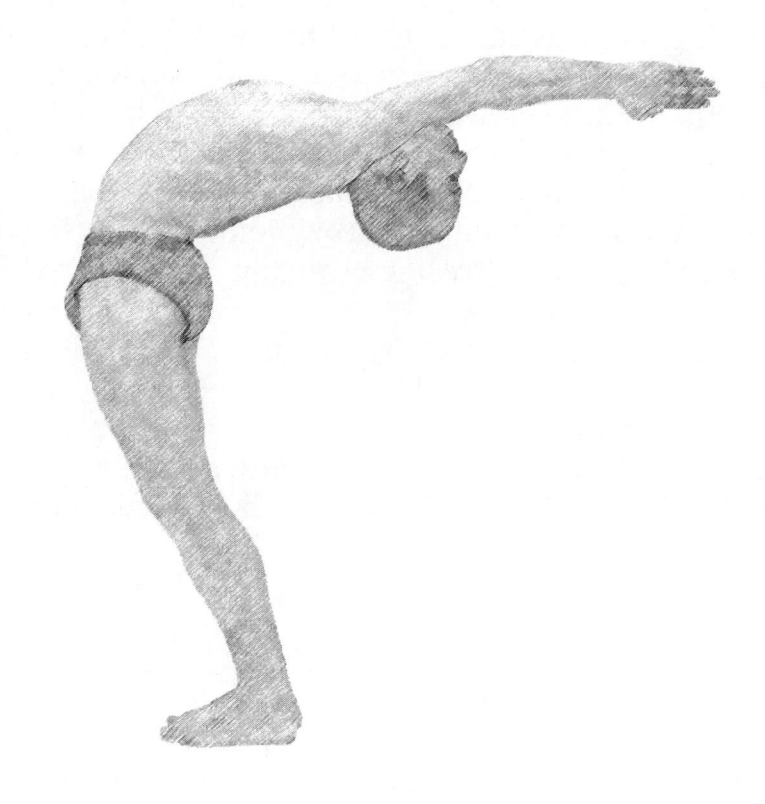

BACK STRETCH

3. BACK STRETCH
Technique

1. From Central Position with feet together, arms over head. Straighten elbows with palms together or fingers interlaced. Realign body with axis. Keep elbows and knees straight, leg muscles slightly firm.

2. Exhale, relaxing head back along sagittal plane. Stretch from lower back, arching spine. Stretch out as far as possible without forcing or jerking. Lift chest, slowly reaching back using hip flexors to prevent lower back from forcing or straining. Concentrate on effort. Take shallow breaths.

   Note: For a sensitive back or neck, place hands on lower back, fingers on hips, pointing down.

3. Shift weight to center of feet. Stretch back carefully with elbows and legs as straight as possible. Feel stretch in hip flexors, abdominal muscles, chest and throat, and compression in lower and upper back muscles.

4. Hold at least 10 seconds. Return to Central Position, with arms over head to continue.

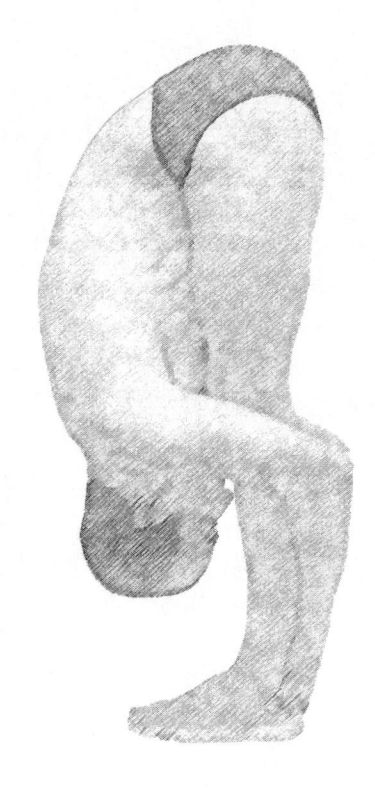

FORWARD STRETCH

4. FORWARD STRETCH, HANDS-TO-FEET
Technique

1. From Central Position with arms over head, stretch upward to straighten legs, arms and spine. Realign body with axis. With chin tucked slightly in, slowly stretch forward and down from hip joints as far as possible, along sagittal plane. Bend knees slightly, relax body, letting it hang without tension. Stretch down, placing hands on floor next to feet.

2. Wiggle hips, bending knees alternately. Grasp heels tightly, bring arms around back of legs to squeeze calves firmly with inner elbows. Keep elbows behind calves throughout posture. Pull abdomen to thighs, chest to knees, face to shins or knees.

3. Work on slowly pushing knees back to straighten legs without jerking or straining. Center weight in front of heels and arches of feet, slowly lifting hips toward ceiling to stretch back and legs simultaneously to improve flexibility.

4. Regulate respiration with slow, deep breaths. Focus exhalation on areas of body stretching to relax muscles and stretch deeper into posture. Hold at least 10 seconds.

5. Return to Central Position with arms stretched out over head, chin to chest to prevent back strain. Roll up to continue into Triangle.

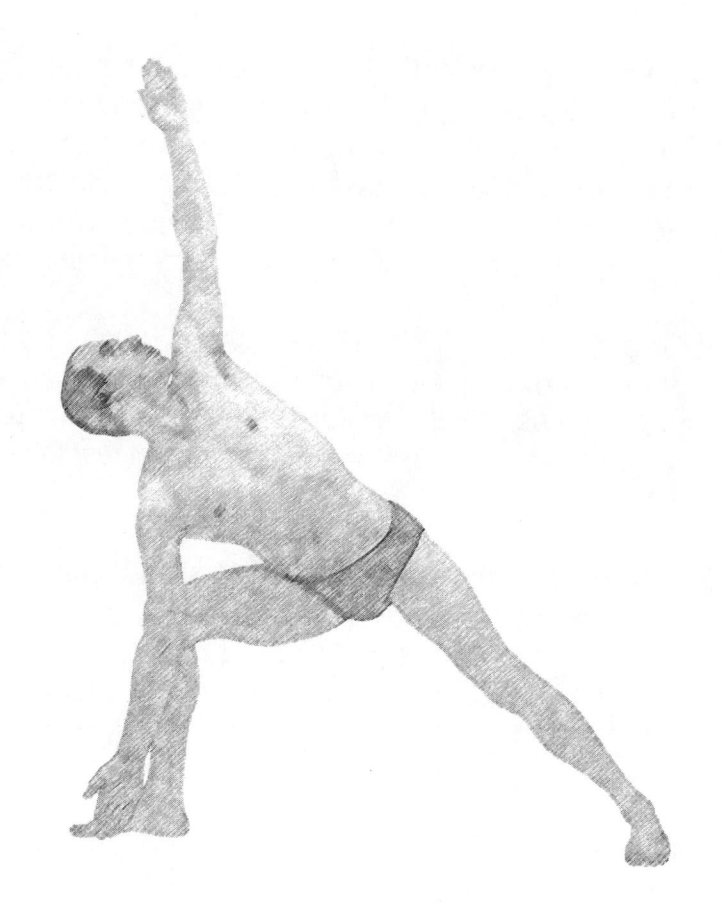

TRIANGLE

5. TRIANGLE
Technique

1. From Central Position with arms over head, realign to axis, step to right, 36 to 48 inches from center. Align feet, legs, hips, torso, head and arms to coronal plane. Lower arms, palms down, parallel to floor. Push hips slightly forward to center, if necessary. Turn right foot 45° to right. Align body with coronal plane. Keep left foot facing forward or slightly in throughout.

2. Bend right knee directly over toes, thigh parallel to floor, calf perpendicular Keep upper body facing forward, hips, torso and legs centered with coronal plane. Notice triangle between right foot, knee and left foot.

3. With spine erect, tilt torso to right from lower back. Press right arm against inside of right knee. Lightly touch fingertips to floor next to big toe, palm facing out. Simultaneously, stretch left arm to ceiling in alignment with right arm. Flatten left side of body. Keep palms facing out, fingers extended and together throughout pose. Turn head up with neck and spine straight. Try to touch chin to shoulder without straining. Concentrate on upper hand.

   Note: For sensitive hips or knees, support torso with elbow on knee.

4. Breathe deeply. Hold at least 10 seconds. *Repeat on left side.* Return to Central Position with legs slightly closer, arms parallel to floor to continue into Standing Separate Leg Head-to-Knee.

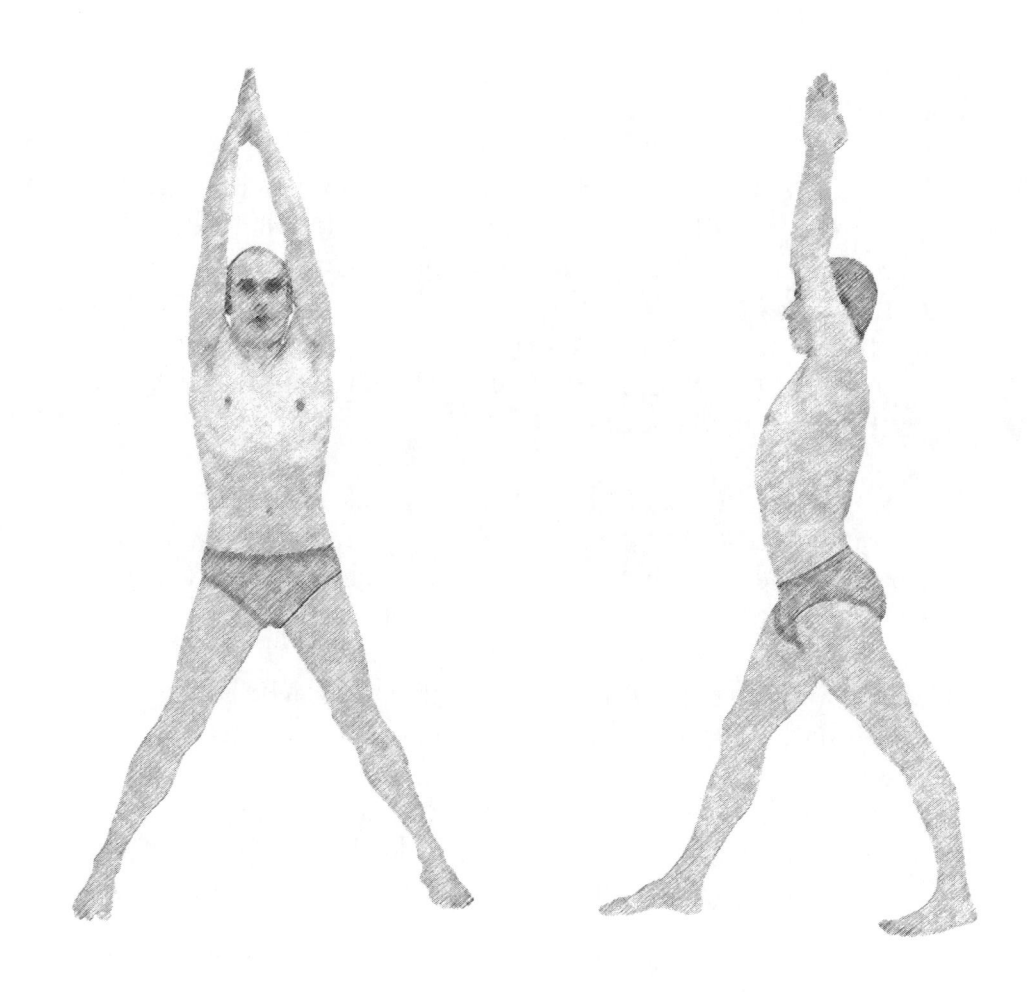

6. STANDING SEPARATE LEG HEAD-TO-KNEE
Technique

1. From Central Position with legs apart and arms parallel, bring palms together over head, arms straight, thumbs crossed. With transverse plane as reference point, rotate right foot, hips, and torso 45° to right, directly over right leg. Straighten back leg with foot slightly turned in to prevent strain on knee from rotation.

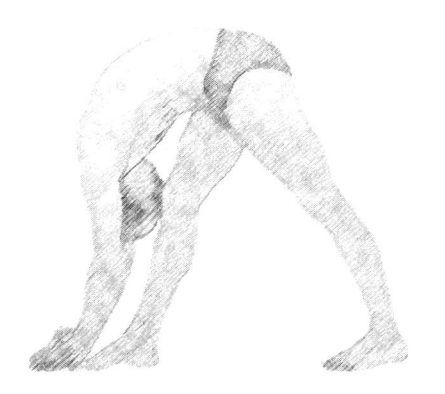

STANDING SEPARATE LEG HEAD-TO-KNEE

2. Tuck chin to chest, rounding spine to bend over right leg. Touch forehead to knee, side of hands on foot, or floor.

   Note: Bend knee slightly, if difficult.

3. Press down firmly with side of hands to help round spine as much as possible. Push forehead against knee. Square hips. Gradually straighten leg.

   Note: If balance is difficult, place palms down on sides of foot before pushing forehead against knee.

4. Focus on compression of abdominal muscles on exhalation. Hold at least 10 seconds. Roll up. *Repeat on left side.*

   Note: Stretch torso up in a straight line before turning to face forward.

5. Return to Central Position, stretching up before bringing arms down and legs together. *Repeat Half Moon Series.*

Practice

AWKWARD SERIES

*Awkward, Eagle, Standing Head to Knee,
Standing Bow, Balancing Stick,
Splits in the Air, Standing Separate Leg Stretching, Tree*

This is one of the most effective series for the development of concentration. It also improves flexibility, strength, and muscle tone in the arms, legs, back and abdominal muscles. Concentration is needed, basically, for every thing we do in life, if we want good results.

There are 10 poses in the awkward series, classified as cultural. They develop physical and mental fitness. It is important to progress gradually, increasing the intensity and effort in the poses slowly to prevent injury.

The ability to master these poses is based on consistent practice, concentration and balance. Standing on one foot in alignment, stretching to your maximum potential without straining or falling is balance. It requires total concentration, or mental focus, on one point in front throughout the pose. Use this point as a reference for alignment and weight distribution.

A suggestion for maintaining balance and alignment: Stand in the Central Position, aligned with the body's axis Imagine the plane moving in a straight line out to your point of focus. The line is the sagittal plane, that divides the body in left and right halves, a reference to realign and center the body.

The postures are usually easier on one side than the other because of the way your body has been developed by habits of posture, work and, even, sports. If you are right handed poses that require strength are easier than poses requiring flexibility on the right, and vice versa.

Physical fitness is a personal matter that needs to be assessed individually. The intensity and focus of your workout should vary according to your needs on an overall assessment and on a daily basis.

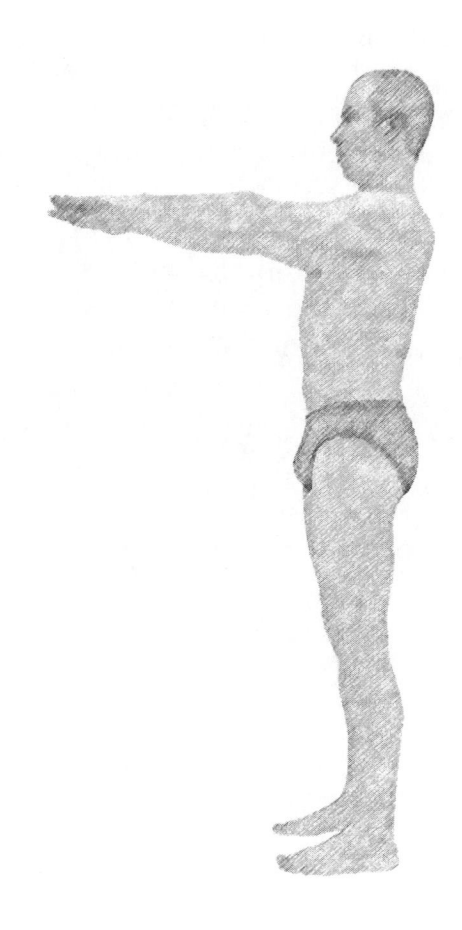

6. (a) AWKWARD
Technique

1. From Central Position, separate feet, a shoulder-width apart. Lift arms straight out in front, parallel to floor and each other, palms down, fingers and thumbs together. Feet straight and parallel, shoulder-width apart.

2. Push tail bone back slightly, bend knees and lower hips until thighs are parallel to floor or, as close as possible without straining.

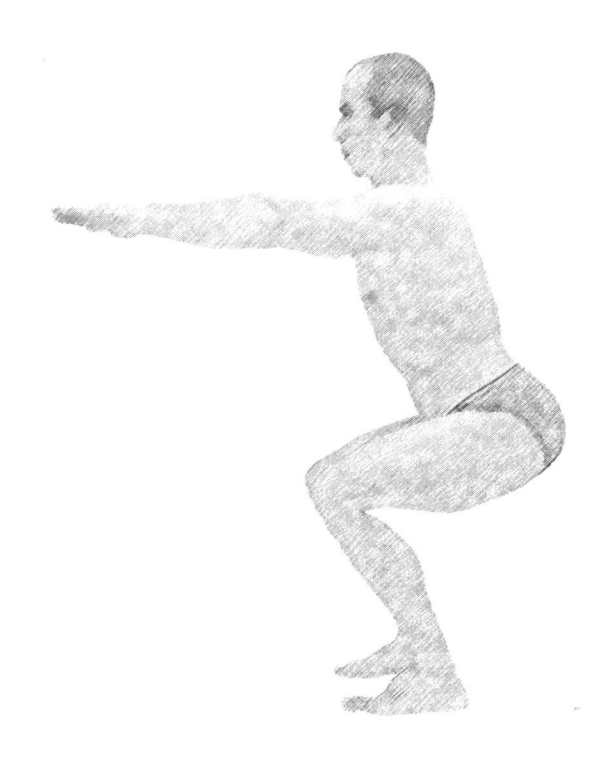

AWKWARD (a)

3. Straighten spine and back by lifting chest up and tucking sacrum slightly in to flatten lower back. Push upper body and head back towards coronal plane to reach ideal alignment. Keep heels, toes, knees, arms and hands parallel to each other. Gradually shift weight towards heels, keeping toes on floor.

4. Concentrate on one point in front. Realign to coronal plane created with straight line originating from body's axis to a point of focus. Breathe normally. Hold at least 10 seconds. Stand up straight with arms up and feet apart to continue.

Practice

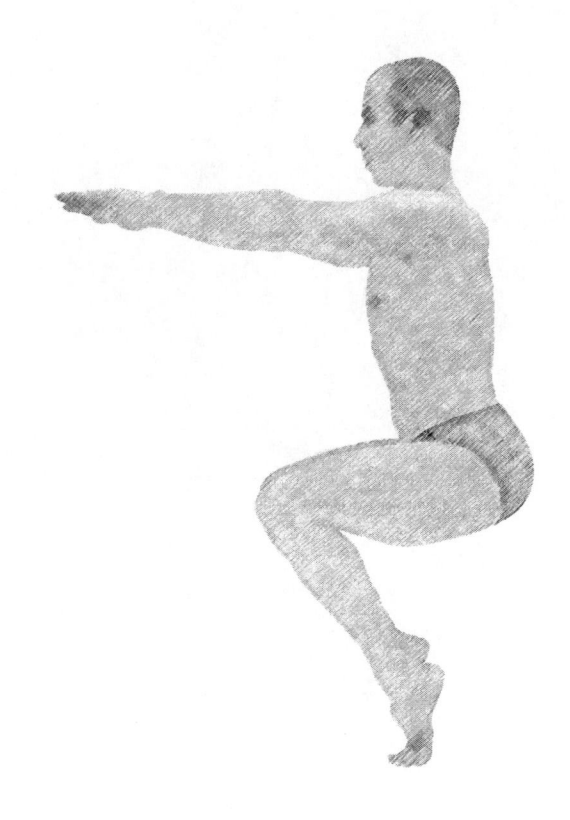

AWKWARD (b)

6. (b) AWKWARD
Technique

1. Rise straight up on toes as high as possible. Keep spine erect, arms and legs firm. Center weight closer to big toes to balance.

2. Align legs to transverse plane. Slowly bend knees, bringing thighs parallel to floor. Keep feet, legs and arms equidistant apart and parallel to each other. Straighten spine and align to coronal plane. Push tail bone slightly in to flatten lower back. Maintain muscles firm in arms, legs and torso.

3. Concentrate on one point in front and align torso to axis line. Breathe normally. Hold at least 10 seconds.

4. Lower heels, keeping arms parallel to floor and continue.

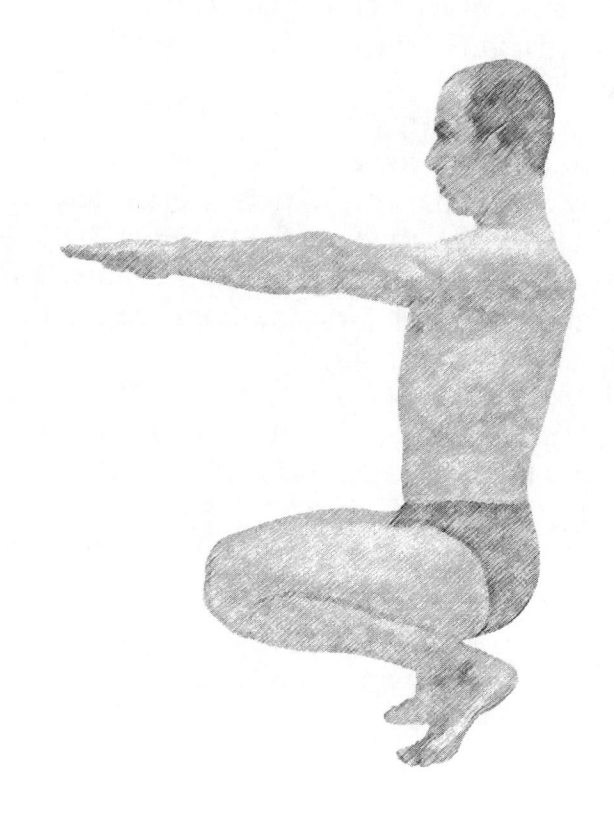

AWKWARD (c)

6. (c) AWKWARD
Technique

1. With feet apart, arms parallel and straight, rise up on balls of feet and bring knees together.

   Note: For sensitive knees, repeat 6.a.

2. Slowly push tail bone back, bending knees to lower hips to heels. Press knees together, center weight to balance. Straighten spine by lifting chest forward. Hold head up, lean slightly back with arms and thighs parallel to floor and each other.

3. Align legs to traverse plane, torso to coronal plane, creating three-sided square with arms, back and legs. Concentrate on one point in front. Breathe deeply. Hold at least 10 seconds.

4. Return to Central Position, lower arms and relax.

7. EAGLE
Technique

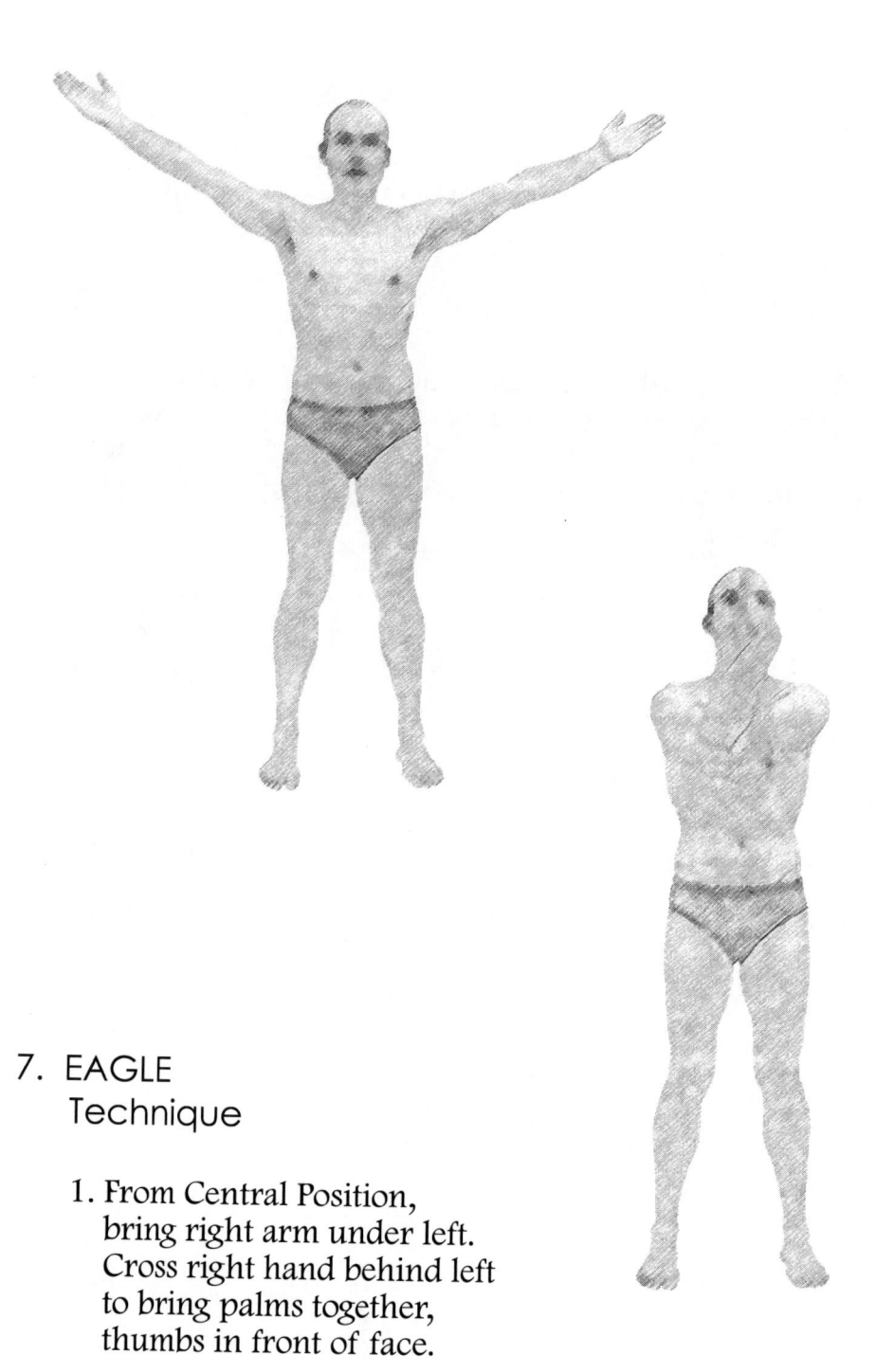

1. From Central Position, bring right arm under left. Cross right hand behind left to bring palms together, thumbs in front of face.

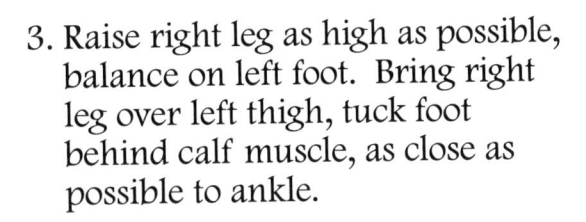

2. Straighten spine, push hips back. Tuck tail bone in slightly, bend knees, shift weight onto left foot.

3. Raise right leg as high as possible, balance on left foot. Bring right leg over left thigh, tuck foot behind calf muscle, as close as possible to ankle.

4. Bend knees deeper to realign shoulders and hips. Keep back straight, focus on one point in front.

5. Level hips and shoulders, align elbows and knees. Without bending forward pull elbows down and in toward navel.

6. Simultaneously, twist arms and legs in opposite directions. Focus attention on pressure created between legs and arms. Keep feet, knees, elbows and hands in one line, hips and shoulders straight and parallel to floor.

7. Breathe normally. Hold at least 10 seconds. *Repeat on left side.* Return to Central Position.

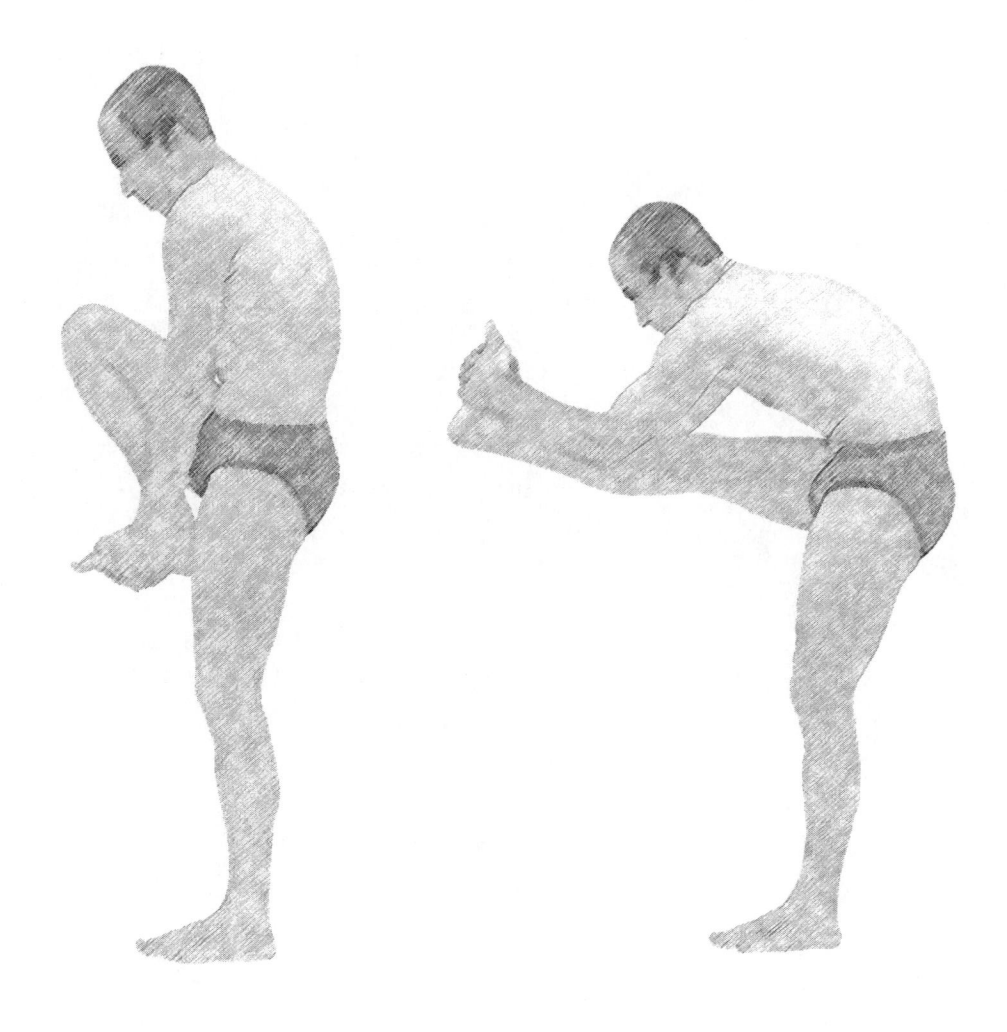

8. STANDING HEAD-TO-KNEE
Technique

1. From Central Position lift right knee toward chest and balance on left foot. Interlace fingers, lean forward and grab ball of right foot firmly with thumbs over toes.

   Note: For sensitive back, lift knee to chest and hold with interlaced fingers. Do not extend leg forward.

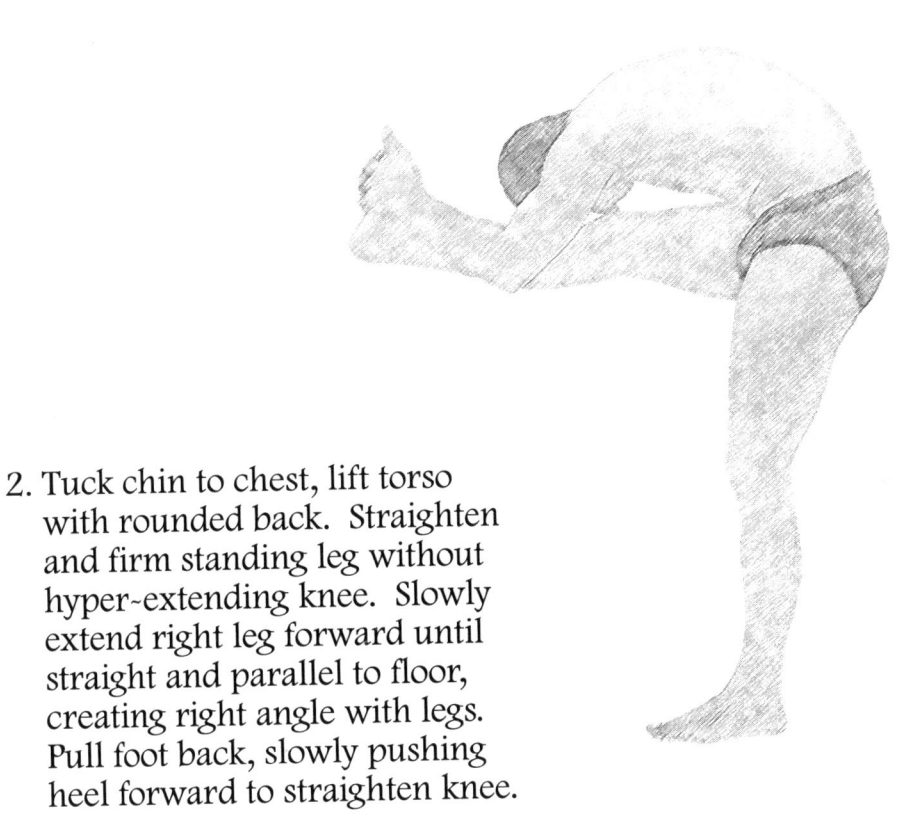

2. Tuck chin to chest, lift torso with rounded back. Straighten and firm standing leg without hyper-extending knee. Slowly extend right leg forward until straight and parallel to floor, creating right angle with legs. Pull foot back, slowly pushing heel forward to straighten knee.

3. Slowly bend elbows down and, if possible, touch arms to sides of calf.

4. Tuck chin to chest, round spine as much as possible. Work toward lowering forehead to knee, pressing elbows against calf muscle.

5. Concentrate on one point. Stretch back muscles and back of legs to maintain right angle with legs, forehead to knee.

6. Breathe deeply. Hold at least 10 seconds. *Repeat on left side.*

7. *Repeat posture.* Return to Central Position.

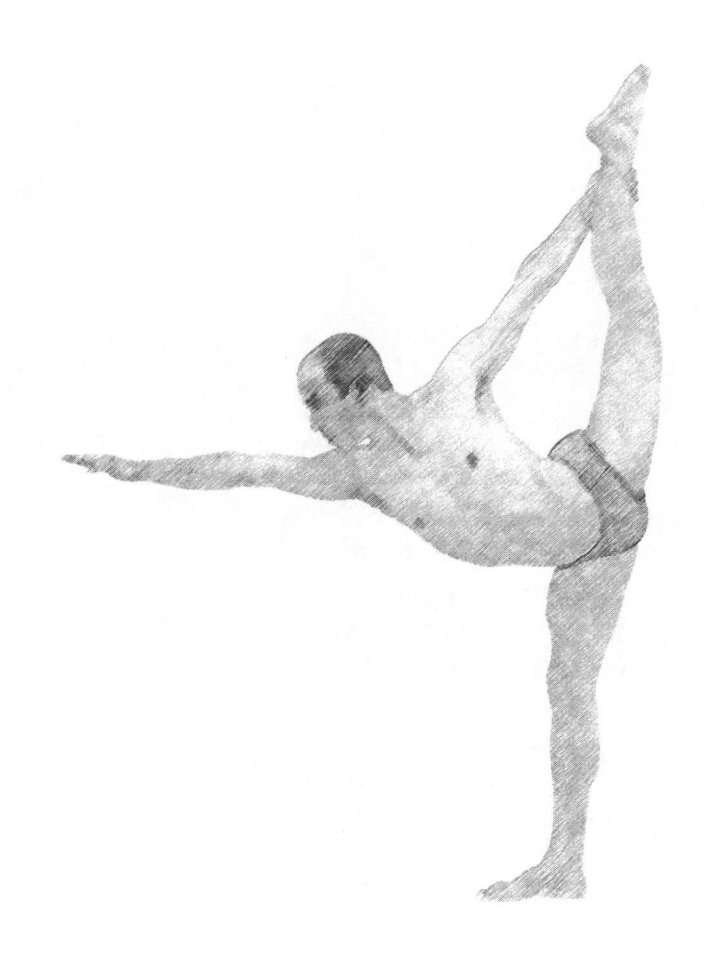

STANDING BOW

9. STANDING BOW
Technique

1. From Central Position, bend right knee, heel toward hip. Balance on left foot, align legs and body with planes. Grasp inner right foot firmly with thumb and fingers together, inner arm and palm facing out, away from body.

2. Stretch left hand toward ceiling, fingers straight and together, palm facing down. Square hips with wall or mirror, lower right knee toward left.

3. Simultaneously, following sagittal plane, stretch right leg back and up, stretching torso forward and downward. Arch spine, lift head, stretch chest forward. Realign body within planes to maintain proper stretching and strengthening of muscles.

4. Work on straightening knees gradually and progressively, always paying close attention to effort. The goal is vertical splits with hips centered and parallel to floor. Asses ability level objectively and work on practice accordingly.

5. Breathe normally. Hold at least 10 seconds. *Repeat on left side.*

6. *Repeat posture.* Return to Central Position.

PRACTICE NOTES

*Modifications * Class Notes * Personal Progress*

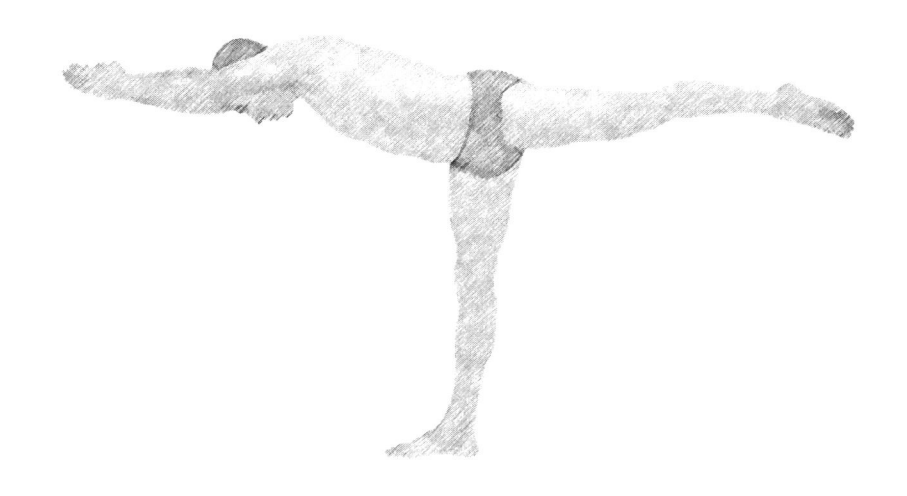

10. BALANCING STICK
Technique

1. From Central Position, raise arms over head, palms together or fingers interlaced with thumbs crossed firmly.

2. Step forward on right foot, straighten and center leg. Transfer weight onto right foot, simultaneously lowering torso and, lifting and stretching left leg back.

3. Keep arms, torso, leg and hips parallel to floor and transverse plane. Stretch body with equal effort in opposite directions from center for greater stability and benefit.

4. Keep standing leg straight without hyper-extending knee. Point toes back on extended leg.

5. Concentrate on one point on floor a few feet in front or hands. Breathe normally. Hold at least 10 seconds. *Repeat on left side.* Return to Central Position.

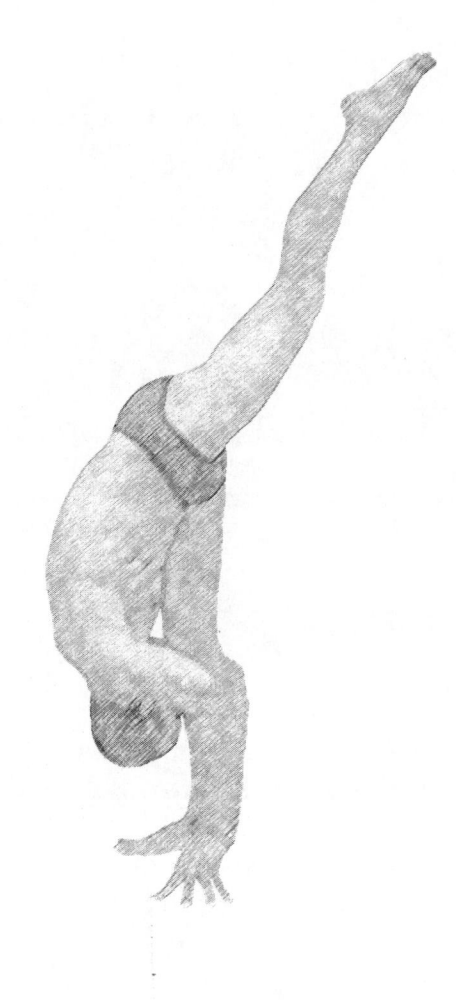

SPLITS-IN-THE-AIR

11. SPLITS-IN-THE-AIR
Technique

1. In Central Position, align body, raise arms over head. Place palms together, cross thumbs, straighten elbows. Stretch up, align with planes.

2. Step forward on right foot. Tuck chin, stretch torso forward and down, lifting left leg toward ceiling. Place hands on floor on each side of foot.

3. Rotate hips down and parallel to floor to align with planes. Grasp heel with right hand, use left hand for support and balance. Bring right elbow around behind right calf muscle, pull body toward standing leg.

4. Pull heel firmly, stretch left leg up. Work on extending both legs with equal effort, upper toes pointing toward ceiling. Align hips, bring forehead to knee. Concentrate on keeping upper foot straight and stretched up.

5. Breathe deeply. Hold at least 10 seconds. *Repeat on left side.* Return to Central Position.

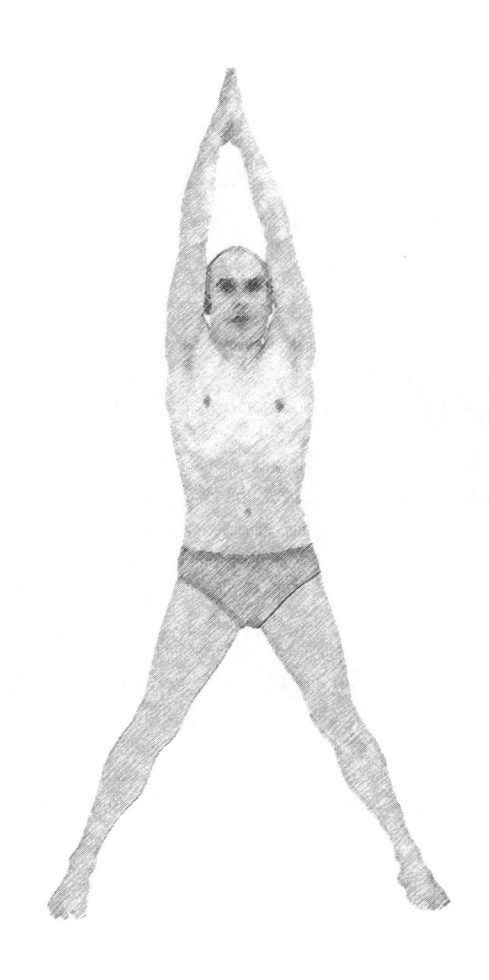

12. SEPARATE-LEG-STRETCHING
Technique

1. From Central Position, bring arms over head, palms together. Take wide step to right, turn toes slightly in.

2. Lower arms, parallel to floor, palms down. Tilt chin slightly toward chest, straighten spine, bend forward and down from hips to firmly grasp outer heels.

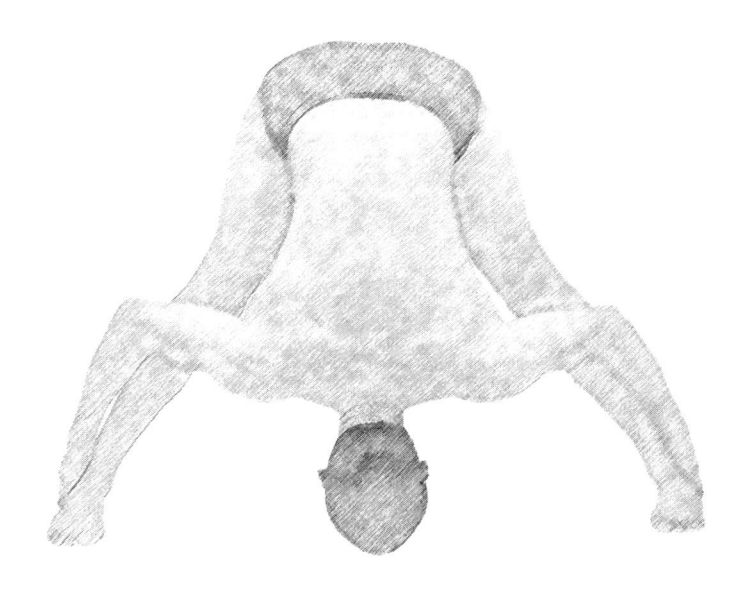

SEPARATE-LEG-STRETCHING

3. Level hips, pull on heels gradually to bring forehead toward floor. Flatten lower back, pulling on heels. Bend elbows bringing them close to legs.

4. Realign hips and legs with planes. Shift weight to front of heels, straighten legs and spine. Touch forehead to floor, if possible. Do not hyperextend knees. Push outward with inner soles of feet.

5. Breathe deeply. Hold at least 10 seconds. Return to Central Position.

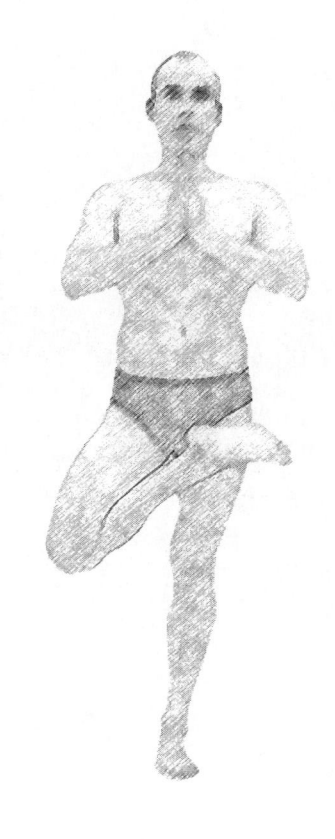

TREE

13. TREE
Technique

1. Align in Central Position. Lift right foot to grasp firmly with both hands. Center weight to balance on left foot.

2. Place outside of right foot as high as possible on upper left thigh, close to groin. Straighten standing leg. Push lifted knee back and down in line with standing knee. Tilting hips forward to align with standing foot and planes.

   Note: For sensitive knees, place sole of foot on inner thigh.

3. Lift and straighten spine, aligning body with coronal plane. Hold side of right foot close to upper thigh with left hand.

4. Bring right hand to chest, palm facing left. When possible, bring palms together in front of chest. The goal is to stand straight, equally divided by the planes and axis.

5. Hold at least 10 seconds *Repeat on left side*. Return to Central Position.

TRANSITION SERIES

Finger-stand, Lotus Warm-up, Shoulder Roll, Pelvic Lift, Corpse, Wind Removing Pose, Sit-up

This is the transition between the standing and floor poses and completes the warm-up portion of this system. Following are the therapeutic or floor poses . They provide great benefits to the internal organs and corresponding systems. Seated or reclined, keep the spine straight and aligned with hips and shoulders, in line with appropriate planes. Keep your weight evenly distributed on both sit-bones and shoulder blades when lying down.

The Finger-Stand develops the arms, thighs and abdomen. The Lotus Warm-up and Shoulder Rolls develop flexibility in the knees and hips, as they tone and strengthen arms and shoulders. The Pelvic Lift tones the upper legs and rear end as it strengthens the lungs, making the process of respiration more efficient.

Circulation is stabilized during Corpse Pose, or Savasana, so the body can metabolize the therapeutic benefits of the poses. The most effective way to benefit from Savasana is to remain fully conscious while letting go physically and mentally. Concentrate on breath and sensations of the body during relaxation to overcome mental distractions. Regulated breath helps to reach greater depths of relaxation. Physical and mental tension accumulated over time in the muscles and in the subconscious will relax. In a state of deep relaxation the mind can reflect on the Self.

The Wind-Removing Pose stimulates and improves flexibility in the shoulders, elbows, knees and hip joints. It also stimulates and massages abdominal organs and muscles to improve circulation and expel air and toxins from the digestive tract.

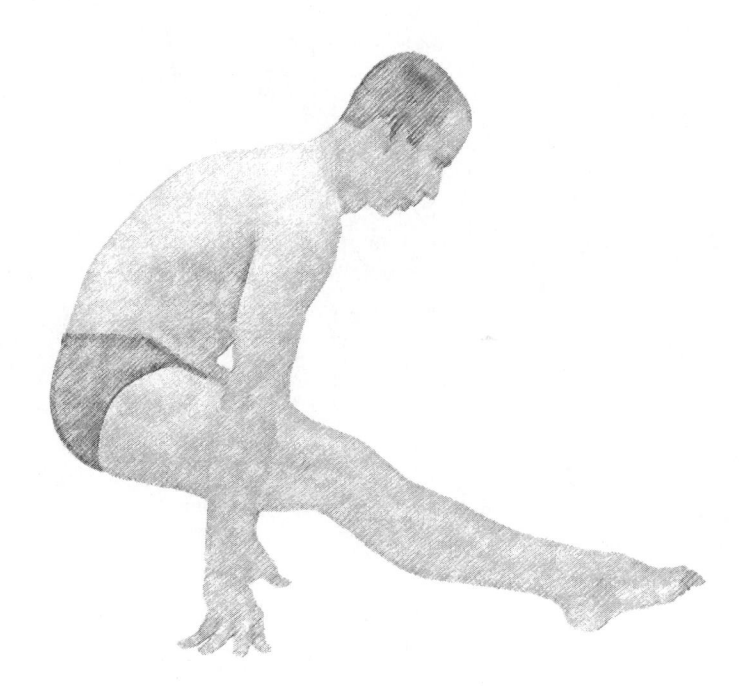

14. FINGER-STAND
Technique

1. In seated Central Position, with legs extended forward, feet together, place hands beside hips, thumbs facing in, fingers facing out. Point toes, tighten leg muscles, and inhale.

2. On fingertips, push straight down, evenly against floor to raise hips as high as possible. With heels on floor, concentrate on toes, slowly pushing hips back and up, between arms.

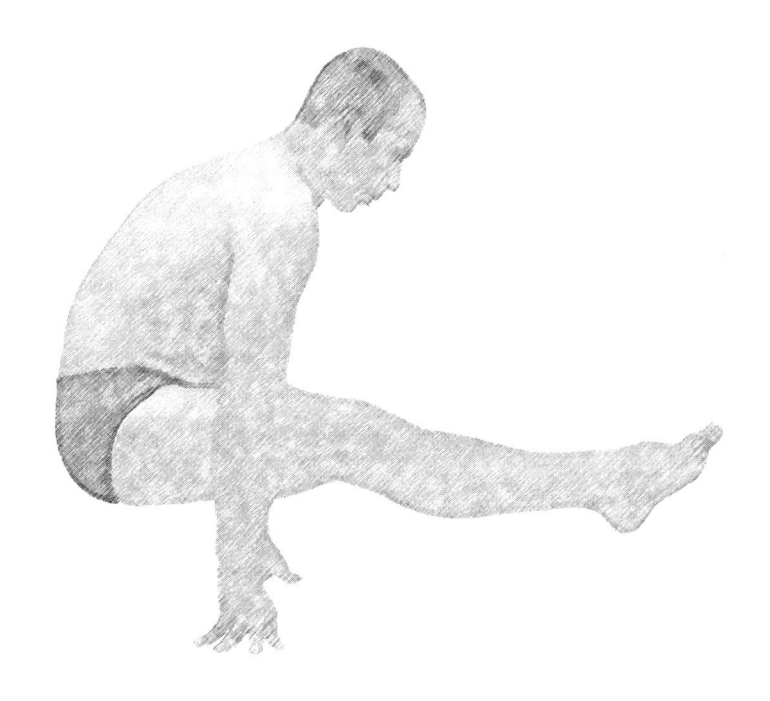

FINGER-STAND

3. With hips back and up, slowly and carefully lift feet off floor without bending knees. Keep legs up, straight and parallel to floor.

   Note: If wrists are weak or injured, keep palms flat on floor, fingers facing forward. Lift hips only until wrist, arm and abdominal muscles develop.

4. Realign body with planes. Hold 10 seconds. Return to Central Position.

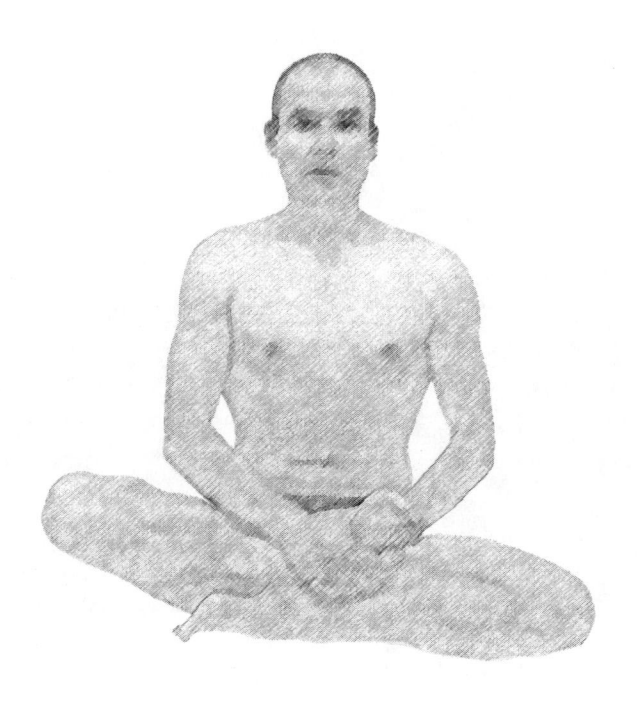

15. LOTUS WARM-UP
Technique

1. From seated Central Position, cross legs, interlace fingers around right foot.

2. Straighten spine to align with planes, shift weight, evenly distributed, slightly forward. Pull right foot in towards lower abdomen, up and around. Straighten arms, engaging biceps and triceps evenly. Rotate in clockwise circular motion 20 times. *Repeat on left leg.* Return to seated Central Position.

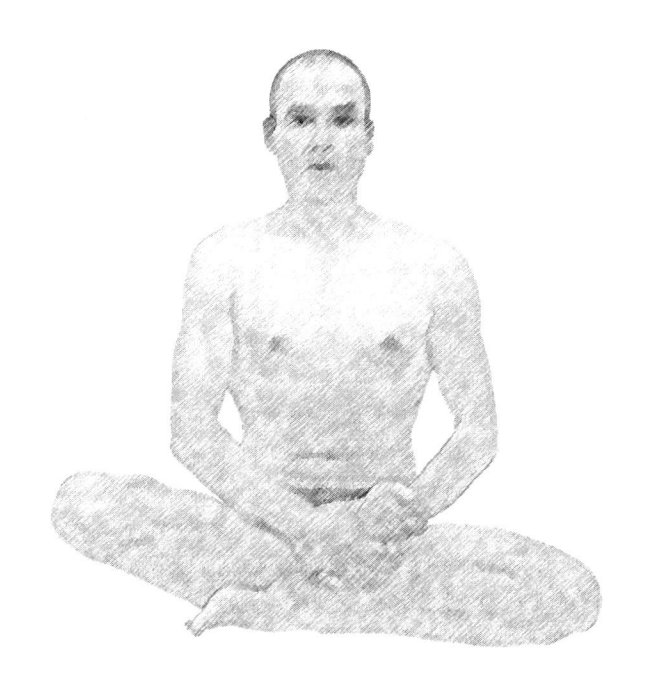

LOTUS WARM-UP

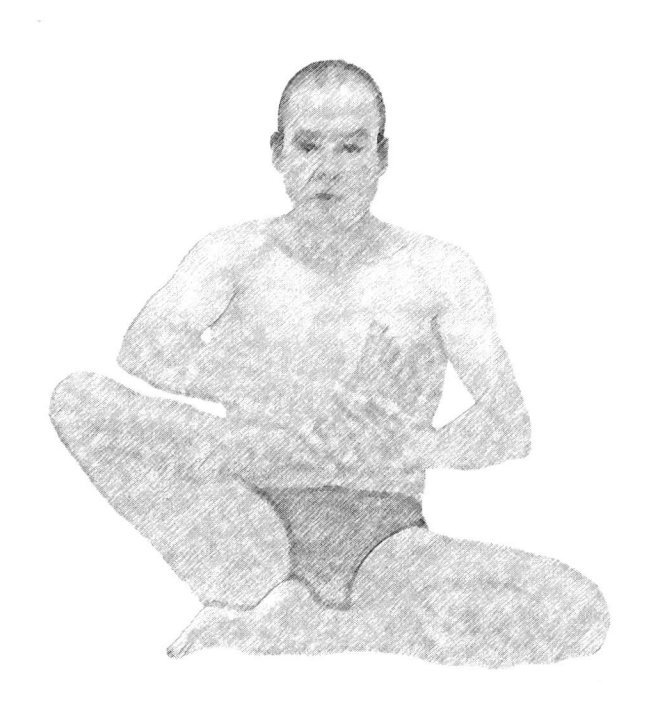

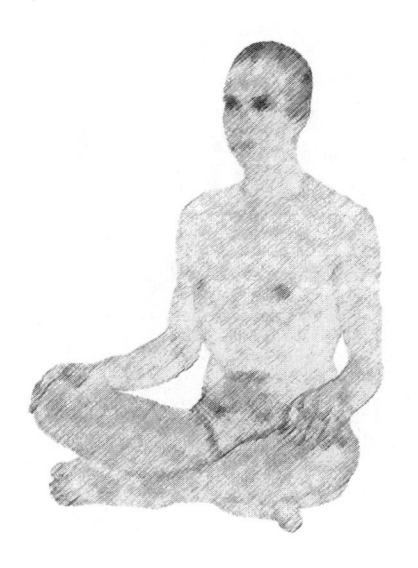

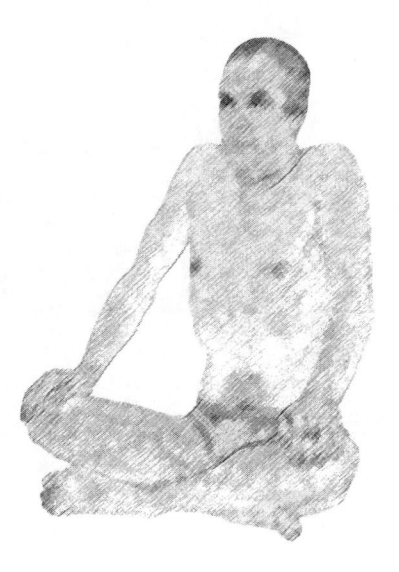

16. SHOULDER ROLL
Technique

1. From seated Central Position, legs crossed, spine straight, palms resting on knees. Relax shoulders slightly forward, then push up with deep inhalation.

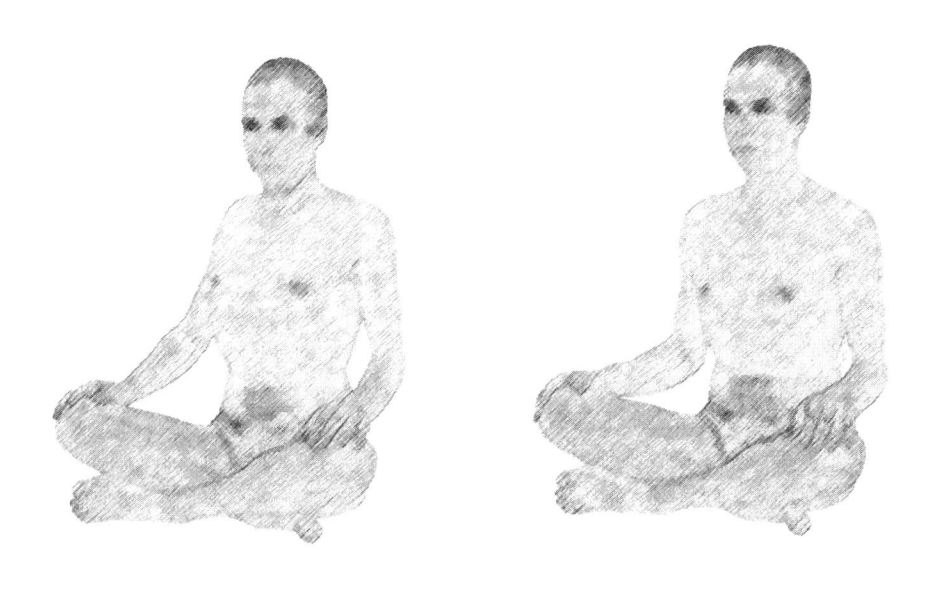

SHOULDER ROLL

2. Push shoulders back, pause, and relax to normal position with exhale, aligning with planes. Continue circular motion 10 consecutive times. Relax.

Practice

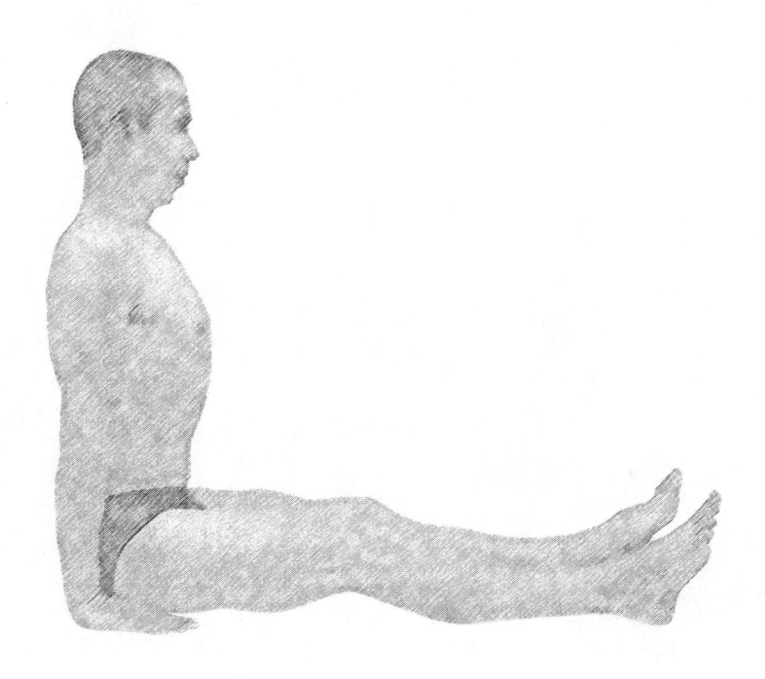

17. PELVIC LIFT
   Technique

   1. In Central Position, extend legs out straight, feet approximately six inches apart. Place palms flat on floor next to hips, fingers pointing towards toes.

   2. Focus on one point in front. Inhale deeply, firming arm, back and leg muscles. Pause, slowly exhale, tucking chin to chest.

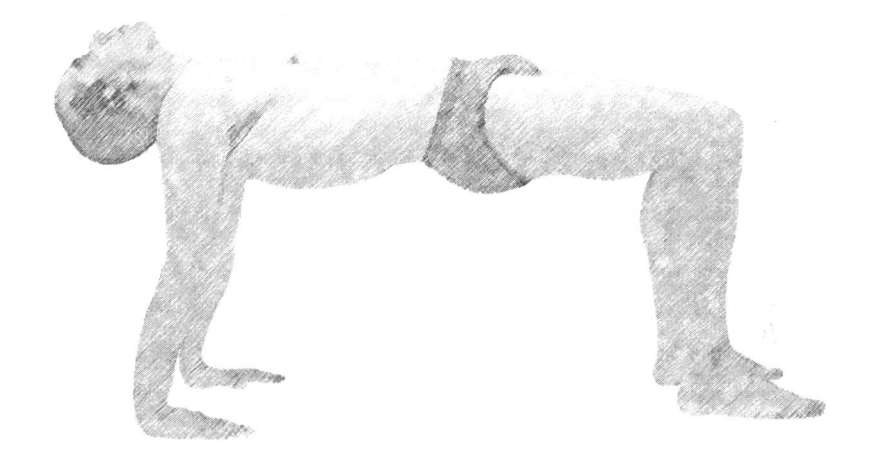

PELVIC LIFT

3. Inhale slowly and deeply, rolling feet forward, raising thighs, hips and back, parallel to floor. Realign body with planes, relax head back, lightly contract leg, hip, buttock and arm muscles. Hold breath five seconds. Increase time gradually without straining.

4. Exhale slowly, rolling back onto heels, lowering and pushing hips back between hands to starting point.

5. *Repeat three times.* Relax in savasana.

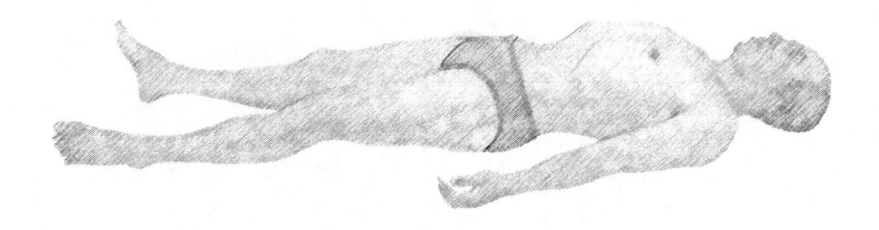

18. CORPSE
SAVASANA
Technique

1. Lie, face up, spine and legs aligned, heels a few inches apart, arms to sides, palms up, hands relaxed.

2. Relax the body systematically. Start with head, face, shoulders and so on down to toes. Feel body parts touch the floor. Sink into relaxation without physical or mental resistance.

3. Focus complete attention on heart and breath. Breathe normally. Relax one minute.

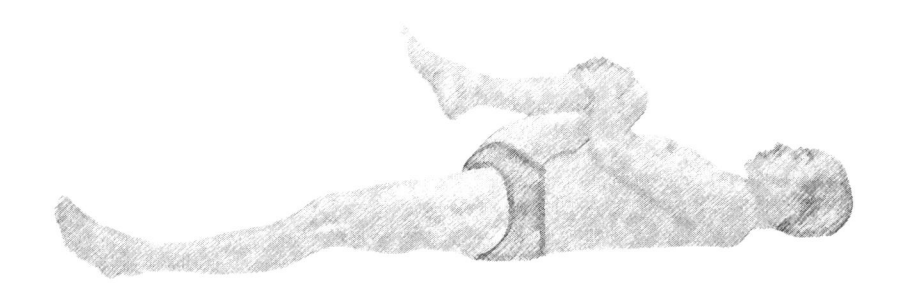

19.(a) WIND REMOVING
   Technique

1. From savasana, lift right knee to chest. Interlace fingers around right leg, about two inches below knee. Touch elbows to rib cage, tuck chin into chest, flatten neck and shoulder blades to floor.

2. Pull right leg down firmly to chest or right shoulder, push hips and left leg to floor without twisting or turning body.

3. Align head, shoulders and hips with planes, left leg straight, foot slightly flexed.

4. Concentrate on respiration. Hold 10 seconds. *Repeat on left side.* Relax in savasana.

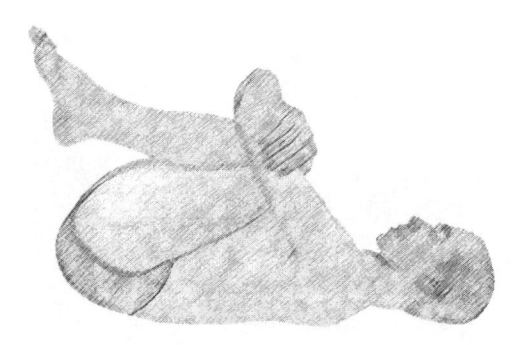

19.(b) WIND REMOVING
Technique

1. From savasana, bring both knees to chest. Wrap arms around legs, grasping opposite elbows firmly. Press neck, shoulder blades and hips onto floor, holding knees firmly.

2. Flatten spine as much as possible without straining. Using planes, realign shoulders and hips. On each exhalation push hips down to floor.

3. Breathe mindfully. Focus on spine flattening to floor. Hold at least 10 seconds.

4. Relax arms to sides, extend legs straight down with feet a few inches apart. Relax 10 seconds.

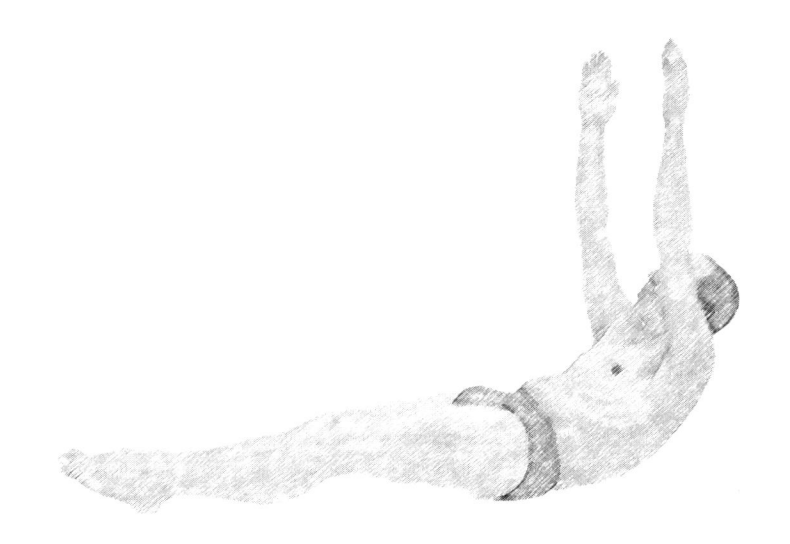

SIT-UP

1. Bring feet together. Firm leg muscles. Inhale, raising arms over head.

2. Exhale. Sit-up quickly with a deeper exhalation, stretching forward twice to touch toes with finger-tips. Turn to lie on abdomen.

   Note: for sensitive backs, roll over and push up on hands and knees.

PRACTICE NOTES

FLOOR ASANAS
(therapeutic postures)

COBRA SERIES

Cobra, Locust, Full Locust, Bow

Alignment is essential to ensure proper stimulation of the abdominal and pelvic organs, muscular development and prevention of injuries. The principle muscles engaged in the Cobra Series are in the neck and, the lower and upper back, along the spinal column. They are attached to tendons originating from the vertebrae, ribs, scapula and skull. These muscles facilitate back bends by contracting around the spine and stretching around the rib cage.

Perform each posture properly, to the best of your ability. The process of mastering these poses is gradual, but consistent with regular practice. Once you understand a posture, focus on alignment and the principle muscles involved. The contracting muscles should support the body evenly.

The Cobra Pose develops strength and flexibility in the spine and back muscles which can help prevent or relieve back aches and menstrual discomfort. It stretches the liver, stomach and spleen which helps improve their functions. At the same time, the Cobra improves body posture by opening up the chest.

Benefits of the Locust Pose are similar to the Cobra, but more effective in the prevention of back and spinal problems. It also improves flexibility in the elbows, which helps to prevent or alleviate tennis elbow. For those who do not play tennis, it also firms-up the buttocks and upper legs.

Benefits of the Full Locust are a combination of Cobra and Locust. It also firms up the abdomen, upper back, buttocks, thighs and arms.

The Bow Pose stimulates the intestines, liver, kidneys and spleen to enhance their functions. This pose revitalizes the central nervous system by improving circulation to the spinal column. It also improves digestion, strengthens abdominal muscles and opens the rib cage, making it easier to breathe.

PRACTICE NOTES

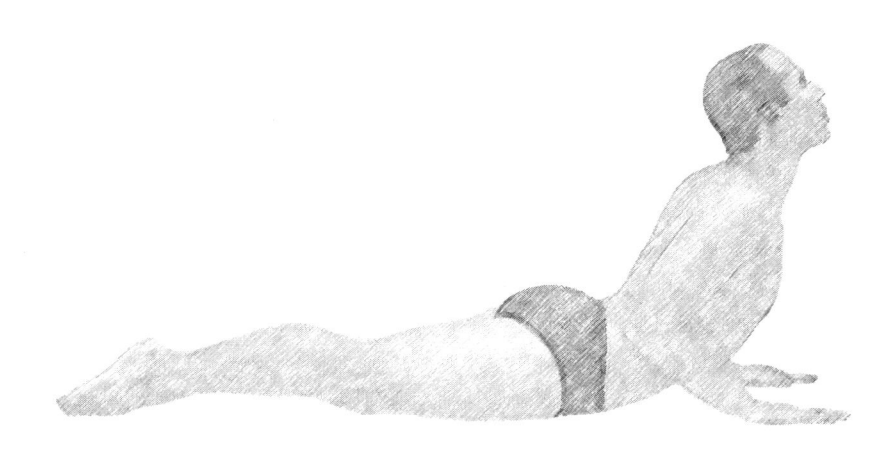

20. COBRA
Technique

1. Lying face down in Central Position, bring legs and feet together, toes pointing back. Place palms flat on floor, next to chest, fingers straight and together, in line with shoulders. Touch elbows to rib cage, shoulders straight and relaxed.

2. Firm leg and hip muscles. Slowly raise head and chest to arch upper spine. Lift torso until navel barely touches floor.

3. Keep feet together and pressed against floor. Realign hips and shoulders with planes. Maintain leg muscles firm throughout pose. Engage back and abdominal muscles to support elevated torso. As muscles develop, reduce weight on hands up to 50%.

4. Focus on proper alignment and movement before concentrating on compression of back muscles. Breathe normally. Hold at least 10 seconds. Relax into savasana, face to one side.

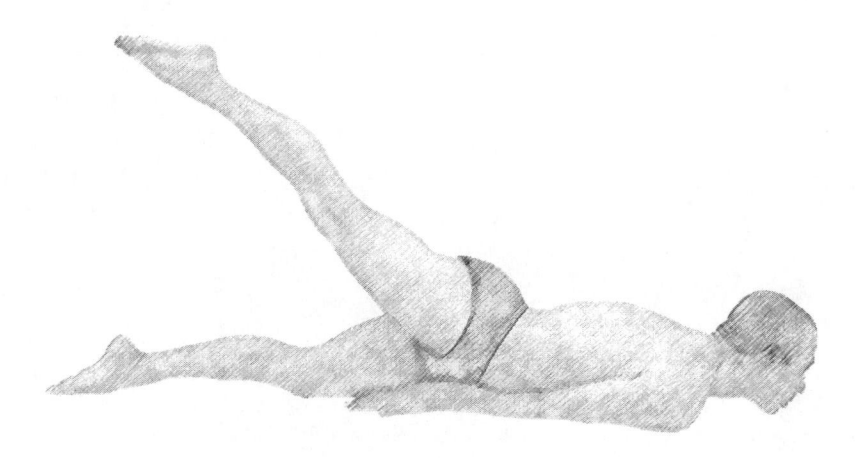

21.(a) LOCUST
Technique

1. From Central Position, bring elbows under abdomen, hands under thighs, palms down, fingers apart. Stretch throat by pushing chin forward on floor.

   Note: If elbows are not comfortable turned up, turn palms up, make fists with hands.

2. Point right toes back, straighten knee, firm leg muscles and lift leg about 20 inches from floor. Maintain hips straight and parallel to floor, in line with planes.

3. Concentrate on aligning neck, arms, hips and leg before focusing on compressed muscles.

4. Regulate breathing. Hold at least 10 seconds. Lower leg straight down with muscles firm. *Repeat with left leg.* Release, face floor to continue.

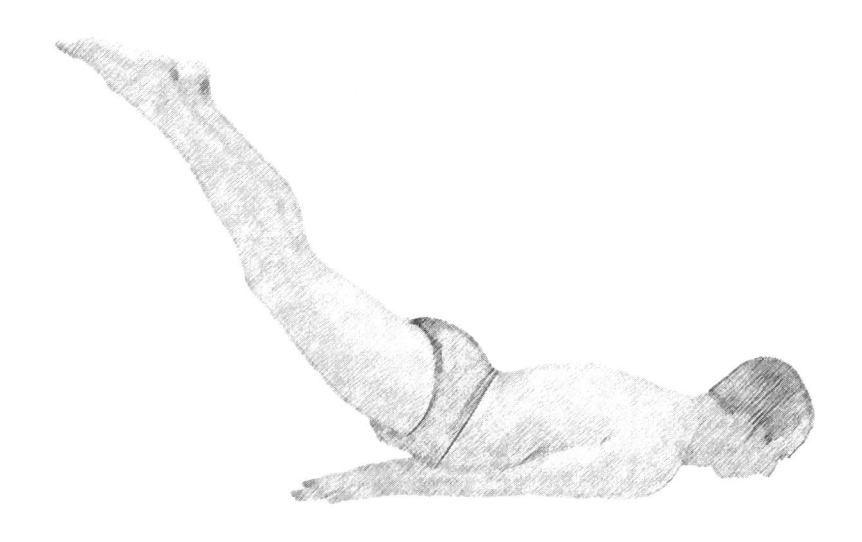

21.(b) LOCUST
Technique

1. From Central Position, arms under torso, palms down, fingers apart, under thighs, *or* palms up, fingers in firm fists. Place mouth to floor, inhale deeply, firm leg muscles, lift together as high as possible. Press mouth and fingertips or fists to floor. Check alignment. Straighten legs with pointed toes.

2. Take shallow breaths. Concentrate on compression of back muscles, lifting legs as high as possible. Hold at least 10 seconds. Lower legs, pull arms from under body to continue.

PRACTICE NOTES

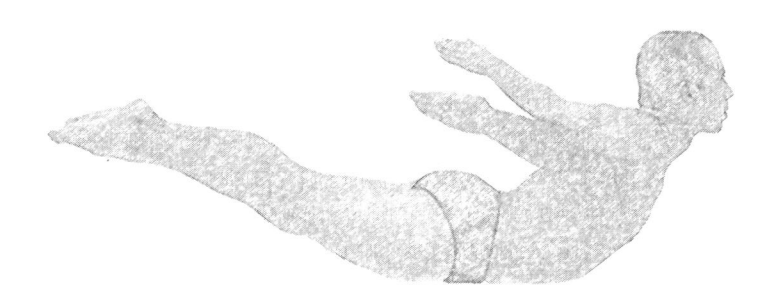

21.(c) FULL LOCUST
Technique

1. In Central Position, stretch throat forward, chin to floor, legs together, toes pointing back. Stretch arms straight out, fingers together, palms down. Realign to planes.

2. Inhale. Slowly lift arms, upper torso and legs as high as possible. Balance on pelvic area evenly.

3. Check alignment. Keep legs straight, firm and together. Lift upper torso slightly higher than feet, arms pushed back, shoulder blades together.

4. Regulate respiration. On each exhalation lift body higher without straining.

5. Hold at least 10 seconds. Concentrate on compression in back muscles. Relax into Central Position.

PRACTICE NOTES

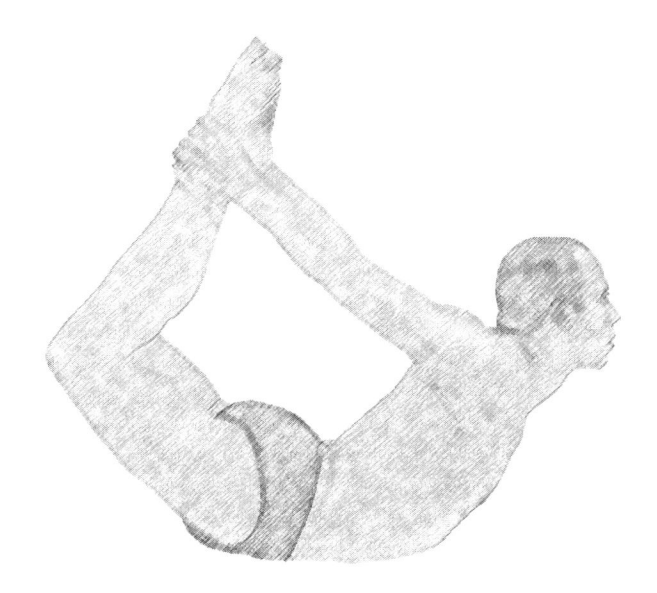

22. BOW
Technique

1. From Central Position, bend knees, bringing feet close to hips. Arch spine, grasp ankles firmly from outside of legs.

2. Point toes toward ceiling. With strength from thighs, push legs and upper body up as high as possible. Check alignment. Keep knees and feet shoulder-width apart.

3. Balance on lower abdominal muscles, close to pelvic area. Look up at one point on upper wall or ceiling. Concentrate on compression of back muscles.

4. Take full breaths. Hold at least 20 seconds. Relax in savasana, 20 seconds, face to one side, arms down, feet close together.

TORTOISE SERIES

Half Tortoise, Camel, Rabbit

The three poses in this series stretch and contract the muscles of the torso. The Half-Tortoise, Camel and Rabbit stimulate the spine, back and abdominal muscles through extension, hyperextension and flexion. The muscles engaged in these alternating movements include the hip flexors, abdominal, spinal and back.

The movements of these poses curl and arch the spinal column gradually and systematically. Compression of the spinal column enhances circulation and nutrition to the spinal nerves as it improves flexibility and strength of the spinal and abdominal muscles.

As strength and flexibility in the abdominal muscles improve, stimulation of the internal organs increases. Thyroid and parathyroid glands that help regulate the organs are also stimulated.

The forward stretch of the spine in the Rabbit Pose is the opposite of the arched-back Camel. It extends the spinal column and back muscles to their fullest as it contracts the throat, chest and abdomen. The compression improves circulation and digestion by massaging and stimulating abdominal organs. The compression of the throat helps to prevent or alleviate colds and sinus problems.

It is important to move slowly and in alignment throughout these postures to prevent injury to the spine. Instructors, encourage students to proceed slowly and not push beyond their own limitations. These postures appear harmless, but can cause someone with a weak spine or back muscles great injury. It is very important to be aware of your students' limitations.

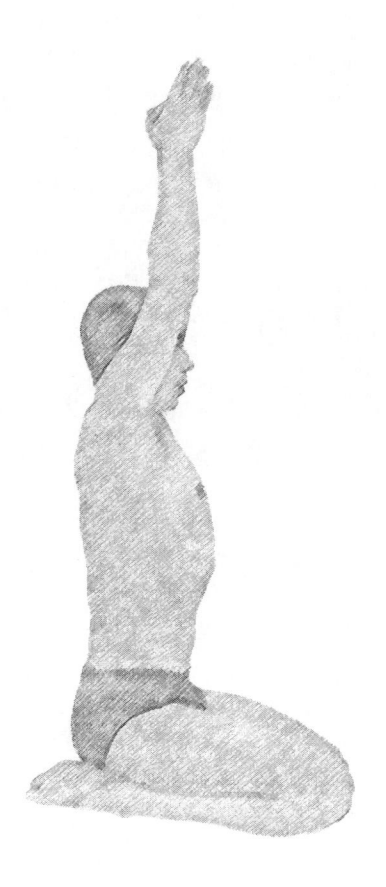

23. HALF TORTOISE
Technique

1. From savasana, push up to kneel and sit on heels, feet extended back, knees and feet together, torso perpendicular to floor. Raise arms over head sideways, touching palms together. Keep arms straight, in line with head and planes.

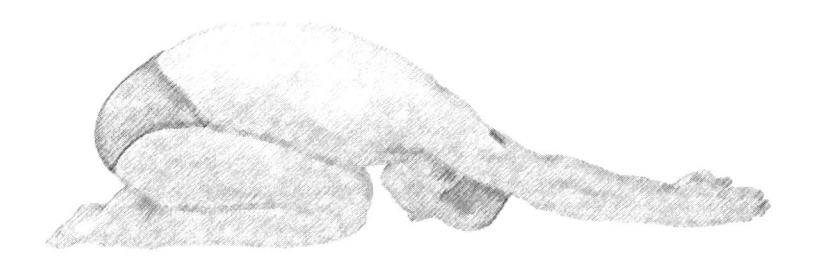

HALF TORTOISE

2. Cross thumbs firmly. Stretch upper body towards ceiling, sitting lightly on heels.

3. Tuck chin slightly in. With spine straight, slowly lower abdomen to thighs, chest to knees, forehead and hands to floor. Keep hips on heels throughout.

4. Straighten and lift elbows before stretching body forward. Regulate breathing. Concentrate on compression of abdominal muscles. Keep eyes open. Hold 20 seconds.

5. Take a deep breath. In alignment, slowly sit-up, lifting arms straight over head, perpendicular to floor. On exhalation, lower arms to sides. Rest in savasana 20 seconds.

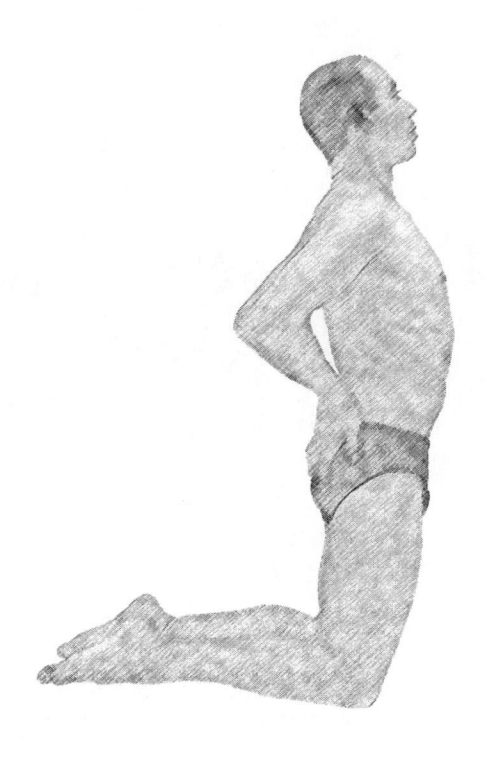

24. CAMEL
Technique

1. From Corpse Pose, raise arms over head, inhale deeply, exhale into Sit-up, touching fingertips to toes on second, deeper exhalation. Kneel down, knees and feet a shoulder-width apart. Place palms on hips, fingertips pointing downward.

2. Slowly relax head back before arching spine, stretching back without straining neck or lower back.

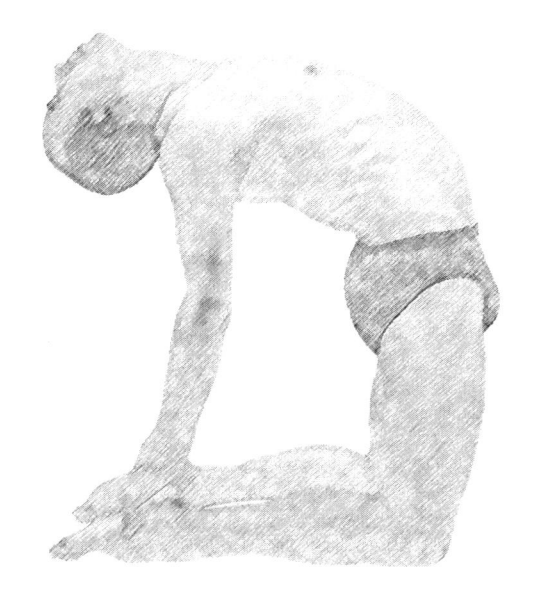

CAMEL

Note: Practitioners with stiff back muscles or existing back problems: DO NOT go beyond this point.

3. Lower right hand to right heel, left hand to left heel, grasping firmly.

4. Push thighs and hips forward, lifting chest and upper spine toward ceiling. Keep head completely relaxed back. Realign hips and torso with planes. Regulate breath.

5. Concentrate on compression of back muscles. Hold 20 seconds.

6. Bring one hand at a time back to hips. Straighten torso perpendicular to floor. Rest on heels then relax, face up in savasana, 20 seconds.

PRACTICE NOTES

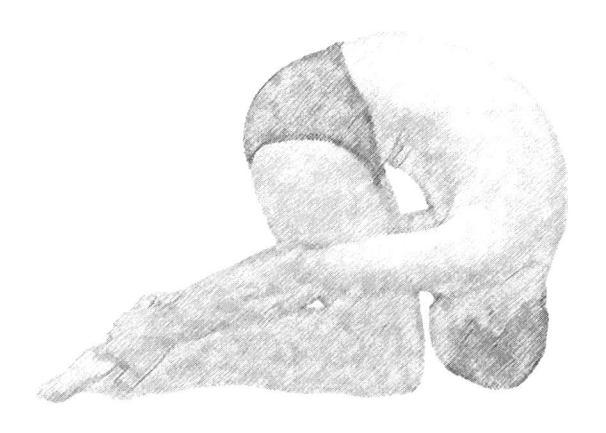

25. RABBIT
Technique

1. From savasana, Sit-up in alignment. Kneel, resting on heels, knees and feet together.

2. Lower forehead to knees, grasp heels firmly, fingers together at arches, thumbs below ankle bone. Place top of head on floor, curling and rounding spine forward.

3. Pull heels firmly, rolling forward. Lift hips straight up, thighs parallel to floor. Curl spine evenly from tailbone to base of head.

4. Keep weight on arms and legs by pressing heels together, pulling firmly with hands. Push shoulders away from head. Keep less than 20% of body weight on head. Realign body with planes.

5. Take shallow breaths. Concentrate on compression of abdominal muscles on exhale. Hold 20 seconds. Uncurl spine slowly, evenly and in alignment to sit straight up. Relax in savasana, 20 seconds.

Practice

STRETCHING SERIES

Head-to-Knee, Stretching, Separate-Leg-Stretching, Upward-Gas-Removing, Upward-Stretching

The primary objective of the five poses in the Stretching Series is to stretch the spine and leg muscles. They stretch all the back and leg muscles while contracting the abs and hip flexors. This movement is flexion. Although the poses are classified as spinal, the main muscles involved are abdominal.

To gain the most benefit from these poses, always contract or stretch the muscles engaged in proper alignment. Concentrate on mastering the poses before focusing on abdominal muscles. It is important to follow the natural movement of your spine, hips, legs and arms to understand and develop strength and flexibility to your fullest potential.

The Head-to-Knee is a very beneficial exercise. It helps to balance sugar levels in the blood, enhances kidney functions and improves digestion. At the same time, it improves flexibility of the sciatic nerves, ankles, knees and hip joints.

The Stretching pose improves circulation to the liver and spleen to help improve their functions. It improves digestion and can help to alleviate diarrhea by improving circulation to the intestines. Regular practice develops flexibility and strength in the upper back and leg muscles, and sciatic nerves.

Separate-Leg-Stretching improves circulation to the pelvic region of the body and flexibility in the leg, hip and back muscles. For women it helps regulate menstrual flow and stimulates the ovaries.

The Upward-Gas-Removing pose has the same benefits as the Gas Removing pose done on your back.

Upward-Stretching stimulates and strengthens the abdominal organs to improve their health. It also strengthens and trims abdominal and thigh muscles, and improves flexibility of leg and back muscles. It can relieve backaches and help prevent or alleviate hernias.

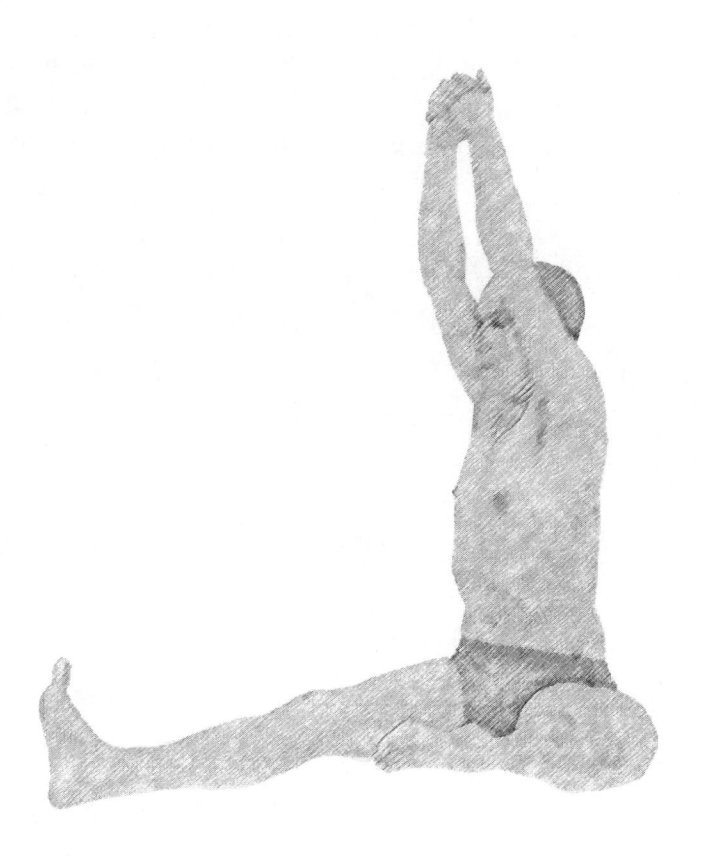

26. HEAD-TO-KNEE
Technique

1. From savasana, Sit-up. From Central Position, legs extended forward, bend left knee to place sole of foot against inner right thigh, heel as close to groin as possible.

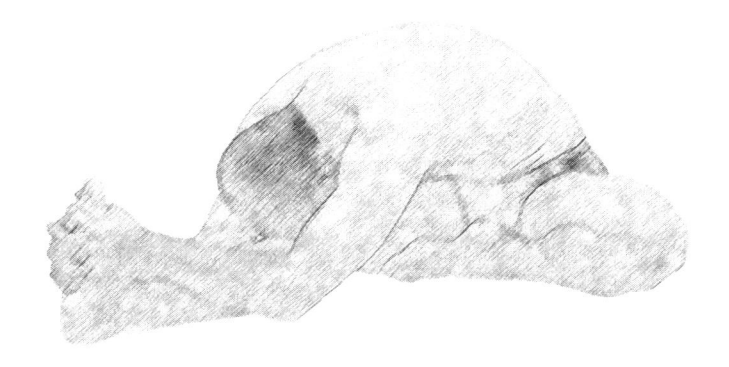

HEAD-TO-KNEE

2. Raise arms over head, interlace fingers. Stretch up, turn to face right foot. Lower chin to chest, round spine, bending forward over leg to grasp ball of foot firmly.

   Note: To modify, bend knee, use strap or towel, to reach foot. Slowly push heel forward, toes back, stretching back of leg.

3. Bring forehead to knee, pull right foot back, bringing elbows in to touch calf muscle. Realign body with planes.

4. Regulate breath. Concentrate on compression of abdominal muscles. Hold 20 seconds.

5. Release foot. Sit up straight, turn to face forward. *Repeat on left side.*

6. Extend both legs straight forward. Lie back in Central Position, pause, Sit-up.

PRACTICE NOTES

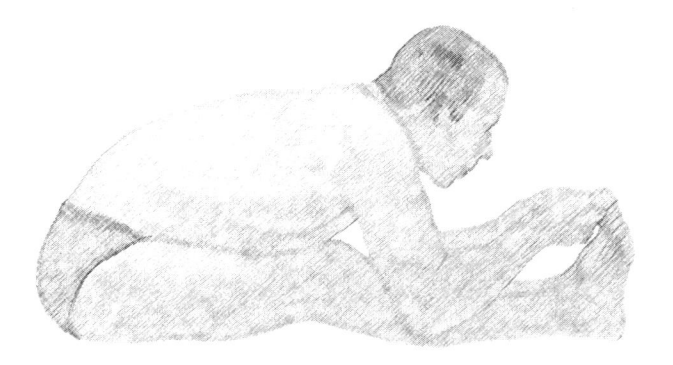

27. STRETCHING
Technique

1. With legs extended forward and together, stretch forward to grasp big toes tightly with index and third fingers.

   Note: To modify, bend knees, use strap or towel, to bring toes closer.

2. Slide hips back alternately to maximize stretch on hamstrings and sciatic nerves. Realign legs and feet to planes, pull toes back, stretching heels forward.

3. Stretch down, chest to knees, forehead to toes. Pull toes back, bending elbows in, close to legs for leverage.

4. Flatten back, straighten knees. Regulate breathing. Concentrate on compression of hip and abdominal muscles. Hold 20 seconds. Release toes, sit up straight to continue.

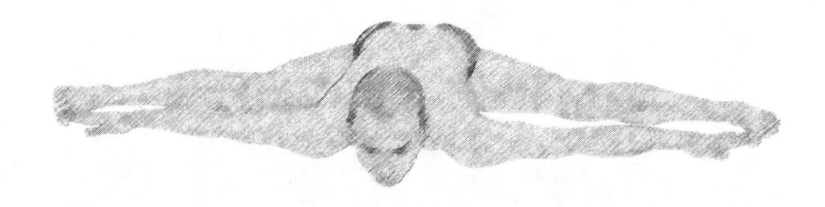

28. SEPARATE-LEG-STRETCHING
Technique

1. From seated Central Position, separate legs as far apart as possible. Stretch torso forward and down to floor, using hands for support.

2. Stretch forward from hips, reaching out to grasp big toes. Roll legs and feet forward. Touch abdomen, chest and chin to floor. Hold 10 seconds.

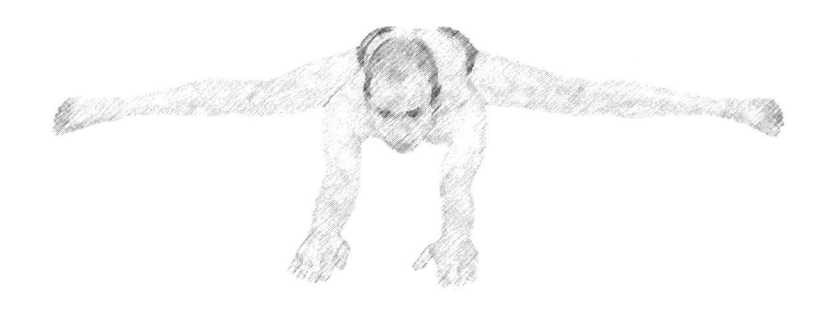

SEPARATE-LEG-STRETCHING

3. Stretch arms forward, palms on floor. Flatten back, stretch forward as far as possible without straining.

4. Regulate breathing. Concentrate on hips and inner legs. Hold 20 seconds. Return to seated Central Position to continue.

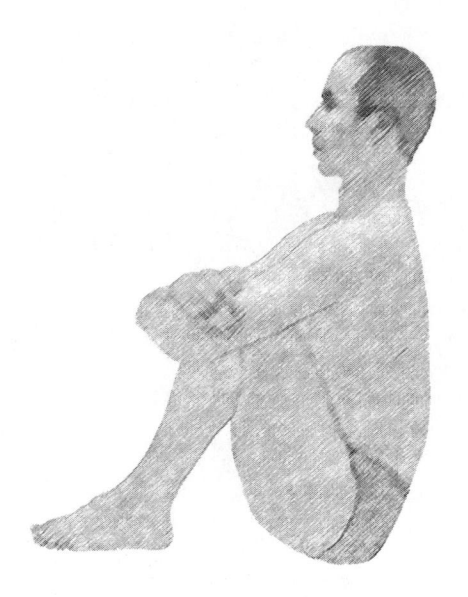

29. UPWARD-GAS-REMOVING
Technique

1. From seated Central Position bring knees to chest. Wrap arms around legs, grasping elbows firmly. Keep arms close to knees, pull legs into chest, straighten spine, aligning to planes.

2. Tuck chin slightly to chest. Regulate breath. Concentrate on compression of abdominal muscles and hip flexors. Hold 10 seconds. Release and continue.

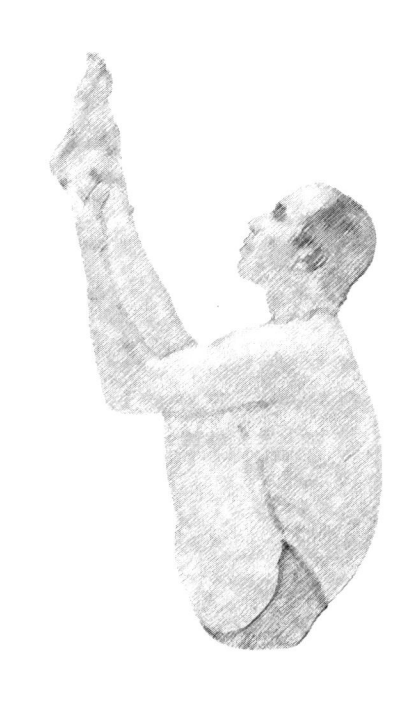

30. UPWARD-STRETCHING
Technique

1. From seated Central Position, grasp heels firmly. With toes pointed, lift feet towards ceiling. Press elbows against calves firmly, pull chest upward, toward knees. Maintain proper alignment with planes.

2. Balance on tail bone. Concentrate on toes. Stretch as far as possible to straighten spine.

3. Regulate breath. Hold 20 seconds. Relax 20 seconds in savasana.

ABDOMINAL SERIES

Postures in the Abdominal Series engage the abdominal muscles and organs to enhance internal and external health. In yoga it is of utmost importance to develop the entire abdominal area properly for efficient breath control and internal purification. Well developed abdominal muscles are necessary to master the meditative poses that require prolonged stillness and concentration. Strong, engaged abdominal muscles keep the organs in their right places so they can function efficiently.

Weak abdominal muscles not only protrude and accentuate fat, they can also cause lordosis in the lumbar region and a forward pelvic displacement. Regular practice of the Abdominal Series strengthens and tones these muscles as it brakes down the accumulation of fat in the abdominal and pelvic areas and enhances circulation.

The poses are divided into trunk-raise, leg-raise and, trunk-and-leg-raise. They are based on flexion of the torso and pelvis which engages the abdominal muscles.

The Abdominal Series strengthens and tones the muscles of the abdomen, hips and upper thighs. Compression of the abdominal muscles during this series stimulates the liver, gall bladder and spleen, enhancing their circulation and functions. Always pay close attention to proper alignment and positioning.

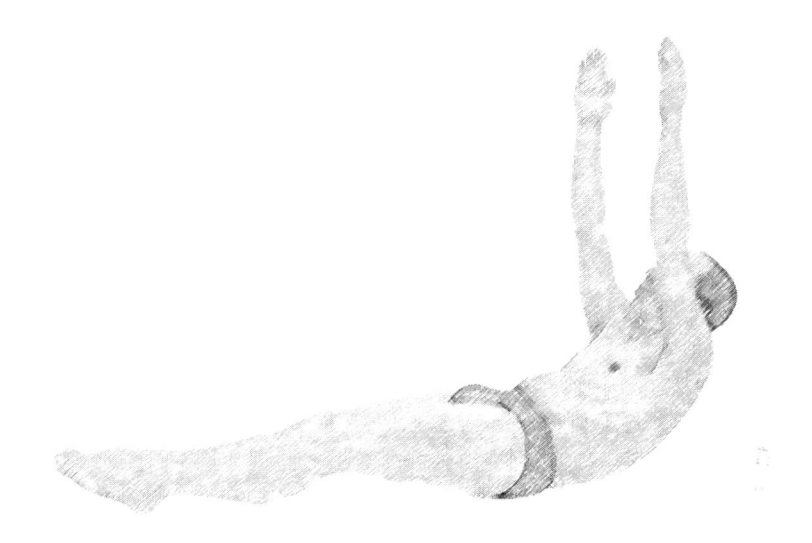

31. Extended Arms - Abdominal Technique

1. From savasana, raise arms parallel, next to ears, palms facing.

2. Point toes, firm leg muscles, inhale deeply. On exhalation raise head, arms and upper body 45°. Round upper back to keep lower back on floor.

   Note: To modify, bend knees, feet flat and parallel on floor. Push lower back to floor, stretching upper back toward ceiling.

3. Realign with planes. Concentrate on compression of abdominal muscles during exhalation. Hold 20 seconds. Release to continue.

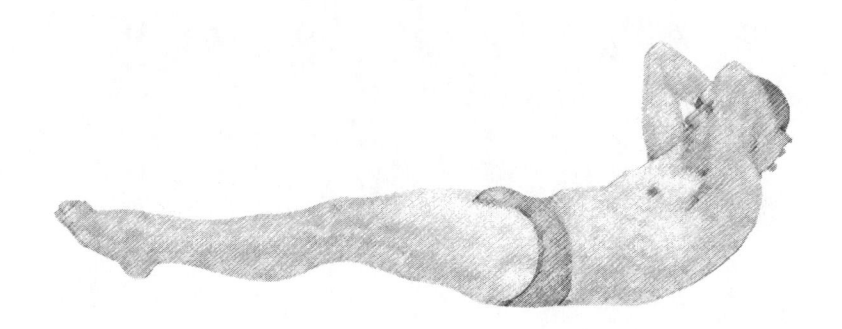

32. INTERLACED FINGERS - ABDOMINAL
Technique

1. Interlace fingers behind head, close to neck. Point toes, firm leg muscles, inhale. Exhale, raising head and upper body 45°.

2. Round upper spine to keep lower spine on floor.

    Note: To modify, bend knees, feet flat and parallel on floor, pushing lower back to floor.

3. Align with planes. Regulate breath. Concentrate on abdominal muscles. Hold 10 seconds. Continue into Crunch - Abdominal.

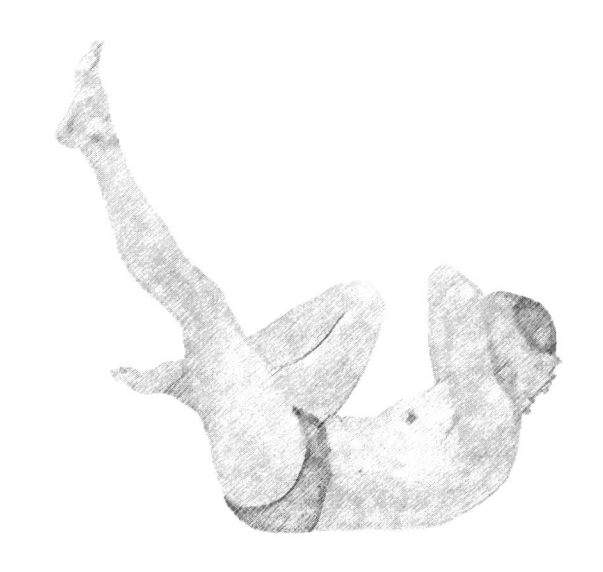

33. CRUNCH - ABDOMINAL
Technique

1. With fingers interlaced behind head and toes pointed, lift feet together 45°. Bend right knee toward elbows.

2. Hold 10 seconds. *Repeat on left side.* Release to continue.

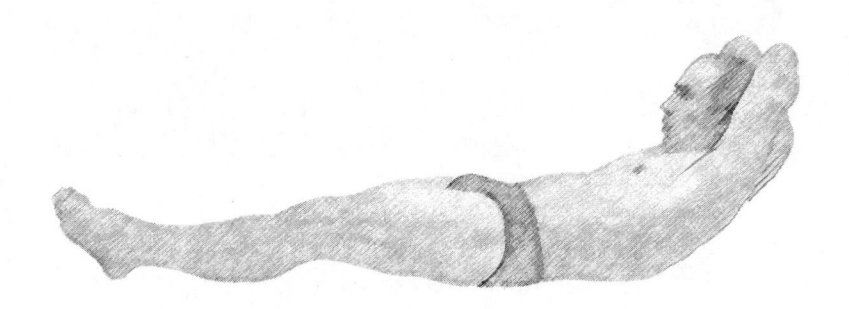

34. CROSSED-ARM - ABDOMINAL
Technique

1. Cross arms behind head, palms on opposite shoulder blades.

2. Point toes, firm leg muscles, raise head and upper body to 45°. Round upper back to keep lower back on floor.

   Note: To modify, bend knees, feet flat and parallel, pushing lower back to floor.

3. Align body with planes. Regulate breath. Concentrate on abdominal muscles. Hold 20 seconds. Release to continue.

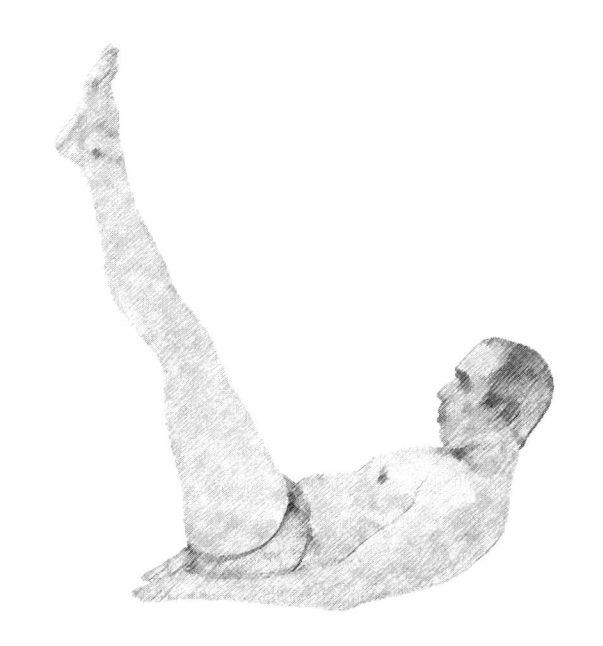

35. ARMS-ON-FLOOR - ABDOMINAL
Technique

1. Extend arms under torso, hands under hips, palms down, fingers apart, fingertips pressing against floor.

2. Point toes, firm leg muscles, raise feet, head and upper spine off floor. Lift legs high enough to keep lower back flat on floor.

3. Realign body to planes. Regulate breath. Concentrate on abdominal muscles. Hold 20 seconds.

4. Relax in savasana, 20 seconds.

Double-Sided Series

Cow Face, Spinal Twist, Lateral Spine Twist, Abdominal Twist

The four postures in the Double Sided Series stimulate and massage the spine, back and abdominal muscles and organs in a twisting motion. Engaged muscles work together in opposites, one side contracting while the other is relaxed or stretched. To maximize development, stretch and compress fully within alignment with the planes.

The health of the spinal muscles is intrinsically related to the health and vitality of the nervous system, abdominal organs and muscles. Generally, healthy spinal muscles indicate an overall, healthy body.

The poses in this series follow the natural twisting movements of the spinal column, the cervical (neck), thoracic (rib cage) and lumbar (lower back) regions. It is important to develop and strengthen the muscles around the neck, in the cervical region, because they support the head, the heaviest part of the body. Muscles in the thoracic and lumbar regions work with the spinal and abdominal muscles to twist the spine. Alignment of the head and neck is essential in these poses.

The Cow Face improves flexibility in the thighs and stimulates circulation in the reproductive system and the pelvic region. It also improves flexibility in the shoulders and shoulder blades as it opens up the chest to enhance breathing.

The Spinal Twist enhances circulation and nutrition to the central nervous system. It also improves flexibility in the hip joints, alleviates stiffness of the spine and improves digestion by stimulating digestive organs.

The Lateral Spine Twist stimulates the liver, spleen and kidneys to improve their functions. It also improves circulation to the spinal nerves and muscles, which can contribute to relief of back aches.

The Abdominal Twist develops and tones the liver, spleen and pancreas, to overcome sluggishness and make them more efficient. It also strengthens the intestines and trims the waistline.

Work on alignment and regulated breathing. Move in and out of the poses carefully, always reversing the steps taken to get into the posture to prevent injuries. Instructors, watch your students' alignment and correct accordingly. Most injuries occur when going into and coming out of the postures.

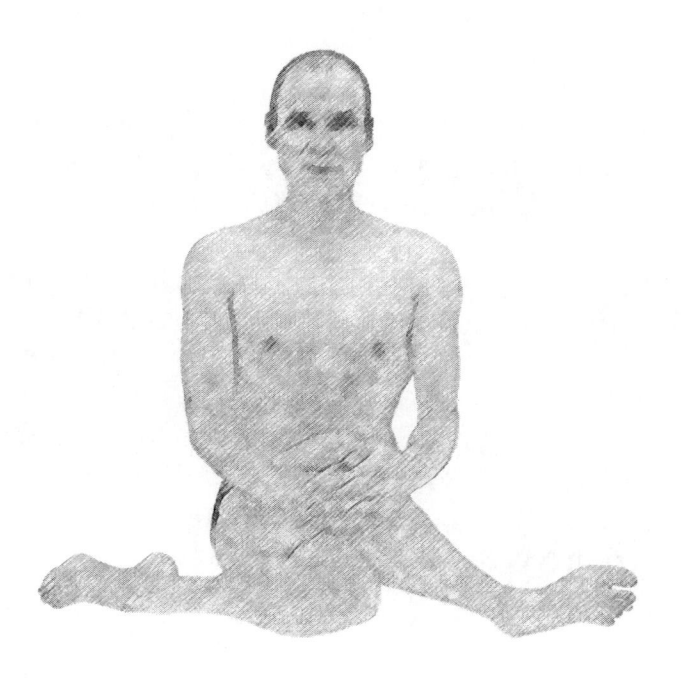

36. COW FACE
Technique

1. From savasana, Sit-up in alignment. Cross right leg over left, bending knees, one over the other, heels next to opposite hips.

   Note: To modify, extend bottom leg straight forward.

2. Close gap between knees, sitting down between heels, weight evenly distributed between sit-bones. Straighten torso, align to planes. Bring right hand over right shoulder, palm in, elbow behind head. Bring left arm back. Bend elbow, palm out, grasping fingertips of opposite hand.

   Note: To modify, use belt or hand towel.

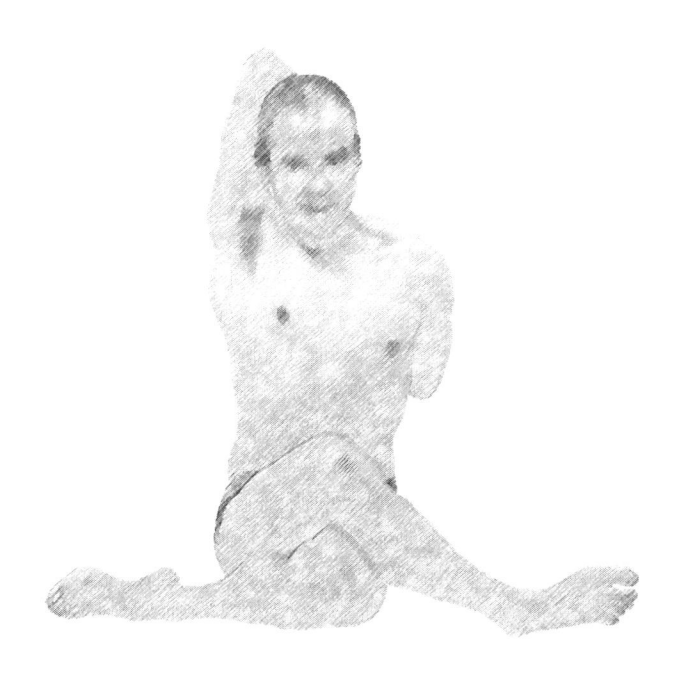

COW FACE

3. Straighten spine, level shoulders and hips, push head against elbow. Pull fingertips in opposite directions, maintaining alignment with planes. Focus on compression in shoulder blades. Hold 20 seconds.
Repeat on left side.

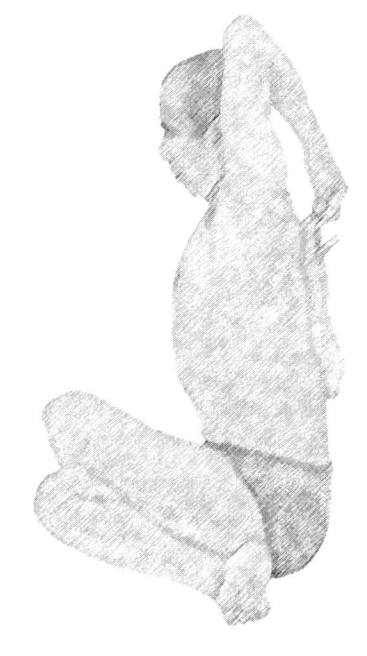

Practice 159

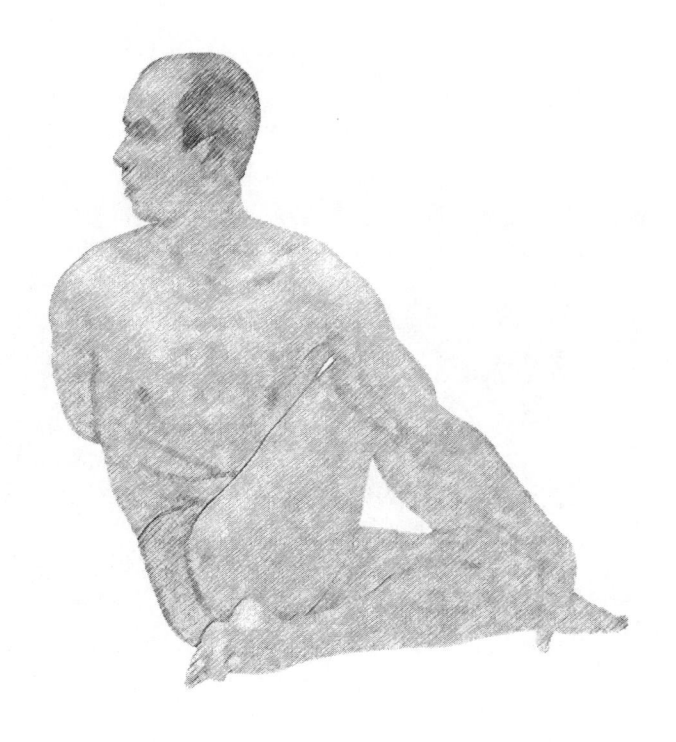

SPINAL TWIST

37. SPINAL TWIST
Technique

1. From seated Central Position, bend left leg under right, touching heel to right hip with toes pointed.

2. Bend right leg over left to place heel next to left knee. Keep right foot flat to floor, pointing forward.

3. Turn torso slightly to right, bringing left arm around right leg, inside arm facing out. Turn left hand from wrist to grasp left knee on floor.

4. Straighten spine, turn torso and head to right. Bring right arm out and around lower back to grasp inner thigh of left leg.

   Note: To modify, sit with legs crossed. Turn torso and head to right as far as possible. Place left hand on right knee, right hand on floor behind for support.

5. Regulate breath. Concentrate on compression of back muscles. Hold 20 seconds. *Repeat on left side.* Return to seated Central Position.

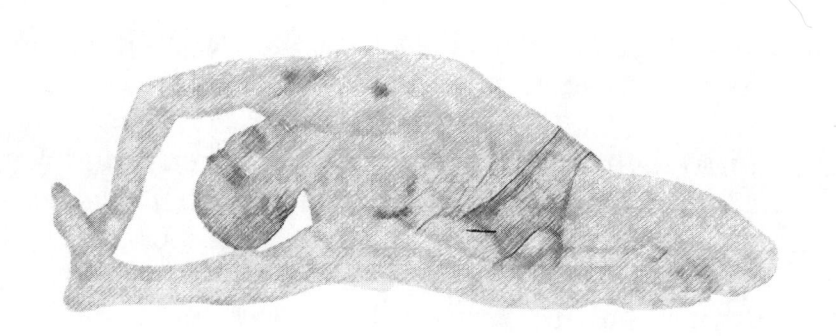

38. LATERAL SPINE TWIST
Technique

1. From seated Central Position, extend right leg to right. Bend left leg to place heel on right inner thigh, close to groin.

2. Lean down to right, placing shoulder in front of right knee. Grasp right foot firmly with right hand.

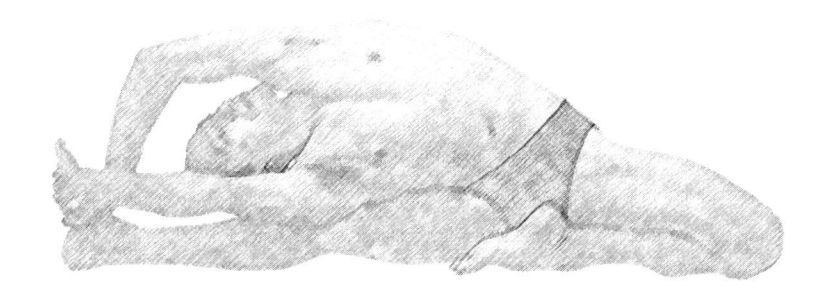

LATERAL SPINE TWIST

3. Pull foot, turn torso and head toward ceiling, bringing left arm over head.

4. Stretch right leg and torso to right as far as possible. Lift chest. Center body with planes. Try to touch back of head to right knee.

6. Regulate breath. Hold 20 seconds. Concentrate on extension of back muscles. Roll torso forward to come out of pose. *Repeat on left side.* Return to Central Position.

PRACTICE NOTES

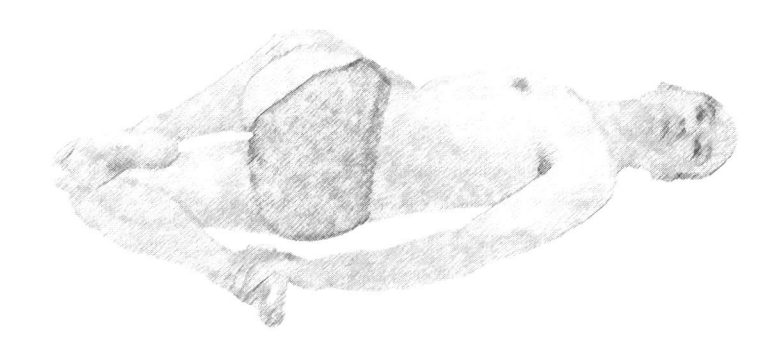

39. ABDOMINAL TWIST
Technique

1. From Central Position, raise right knee toward chest, turn to left side. Place right foot on left inner thigh.

2. Keep shoulder blades flat on floor. Bend left leg back toward right hip. Place left hand on right knee. Grasp left foot with right hand.

3. Resist with right hip, pressing down on right knee with left hand, and left foot with right hand. Turn head and torso to right, shoulder blades and lower back on floor, aligned with planes.

4. Regulate breath. Concentrate on abdominal muscles. Hold 20 seconds. *Repeat on left side.* Relax in savasana, 20 seconds.

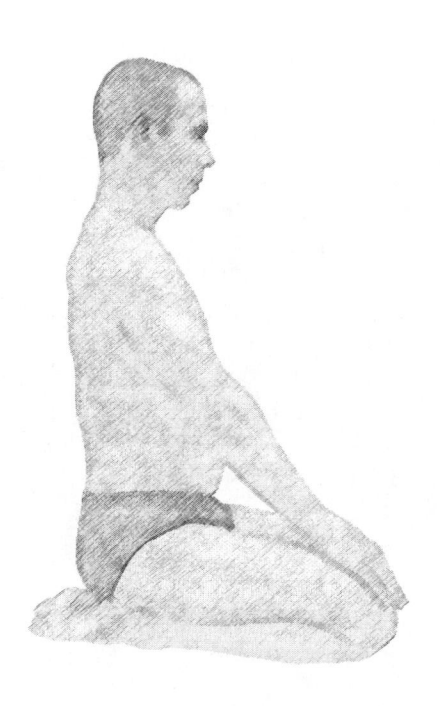

BREATHING SERIES
(part II)

The Blowing Pose, or *Kapalabhati,* is the final exercise. The key to success is in the abdominal muscles functioning like a bellow. This exercise expels stagnant air and toxins from the body. Immediate release of the abdominal muscles after a quick and firm contraction automatically draws air back into your lungs. To prevent shortness of breath, be sure to contract the abdominal muscles quickly and firmly to expel as much air as possible, then quickly release and relax the muscles to draw in as much fresh air as possible.

Prenatal women: DO NOT practice this exercise.

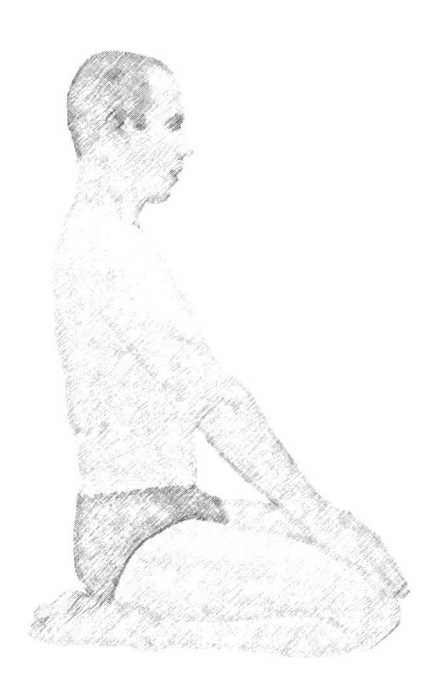

40. BLOWING POSE - *Kapalabhati*
Technique

1. From savasana, Sit-up in alignment. Kneel with sit-bones resting comfortably on back of legs near heels

   Note: To modify, sit crossed-legged, weight evenly distributed, spine and head straight, shoulders and hips parallel, palms on knees.

2. Relax abdominal muscles to inhale then contract quickly and firmly using diaphragm to completely expel air from lungs through mouth as if blowing. Immediately release abdominal muscles to draw fresh air back into lungs.

3. Concentrate on compression of abdomen. Repeat 60 times, pause, repeat. Relax in savasana, at least two minutes.

Final Notes

The *Yoga Challenge® I* is the foundation of the four Yoga Challenge systems. The principles of alignment and practice apply to all. The postures originate from the 84 classic asanas organized by Bishnu Ghosh and Swami Sivananda Saraswati. They are a combination of cultural, meditative and therapeutic postures. The final breathing exercise, kapalabhati, not only cools the body down and expels stagnant air and toxins, it prepares the body for complete relaxation that allows the therapeutic benefits to manifest.

It is important to follow basic principles of practice to prevent injury:

1. Align with planes
2. Distribute weight evenly
3. Move slowly and mindfully
4. Come out of postures in reverse movement
5. Breathe mindfully
6. Practice within your limitations & strengths

"Like an unbaked urn left in water,
the bodily vessel becomes ever so decayed.
Baked well in the fire of Yoga,
the vessel becomes purified and enduring"
Gheranda Samhita

Bibliography

BIBLIOGRAPHY

Ancient Indian Tradition & Mythology, The Shiva Purana, Volume 1,2, 3, translated by a board of scholars, 1970, Motilal Banarsidass Publishers, Delhi, India.

The Bhagavadgita, by Kees Bolle, 1979, University of California Press.

Bikram's Beginning Yoga Class, Bikram Choudhury, 1997, Tarcher/Putnam.

Body Worlds, The Anatomical Exhibition of Real Human Bodies, Gunther Von Hagens.

A Buddhist Bible, edited by Dwight Goddard, 1994, Beacon Press, Boston, USA.

Garuda Puranam, The Chowkhamba Sanskrit Series, Manmathanath Duit Shastri, 1968, Varanasi, India.

The Gods and Their Symbols, Eva Rudy Jansen, 1993, Binkey Kok Publications, Holland.

Gorakhnath and the Kampata Yogis, George Weston Briggs, 1938, Delhi, India.

Great Systems of Yoga, Ernest Wood, 1954, Philosophical Library, New York.

Hatha-Yoga, An Advanced Method of Physical Education and Concentration, Professor Shyam Sundar Goswami, 1963, L.N. Fowler & Co., LTD, London.

The Hatha Yoga Pradipika, translated by Panchm Sinh, 1980, Munshiram Manoharlal Publishers, LTD., New Delhi, India.

Hatha Yoga Pradipika, Light on Hatha Yoga, published by Sri G.K. Kejriwal, 1998, Bihar School of Yoga Munger (Bihar) India.

Kaulajnana Nirnaya of the School of Matsendranatha, P.C. Bagchi, 1986, translated into English by Michael Magge, Prachya Prakashan, Varanasi, India.

Light on Yoga, B.K.S. Iyengar, 1976, George Allen & Unwin LTD.

The Matsyamahapuranam, Vol. 1 & 2, Second Edition 1997, Nag Publishers, Delhi, India.

Muscle Testing and Function, Florence P. Kendall & Elizabeth K. McCreary, 1983, USA.

Personal Fitness, Looking Good/Feeling Good, Charles S. Williams, Emmanuel G. Harageones, Dewayne J. Johnson & Charles D. Smith, 1995, Kendall/Hunt Publishing Co.

Philosophy of Gorakhnath with Goraksha-Vacana-Sangraha, Akshaya Kumar Banerjea, Motilal Banarsidass, 1962, Delhi, Varanasi, Patna, India.

Popular Yoga Asanas, Swami Kuvalayananda, 1972, Charles E. Tuttle Co., Rutland, Vermont & Tokyo.

The Shambhala Encyclopedia of Yoga, Georg Feuerstein PhD, 1997, Boston.

The Yoga System of Patanjali, The Ancient Hindu Doctrine of Concentration of the Mind, Harvard Oriental Series, Vol. 17, James Haughton Woods, 1966, Delhi.

Made in the USA